BRAIN FOOD DIET

COGNITIVE DECLINE AND ALZHEIMER'S DISEASE REVERSED WITH ANTI-AGING LONGEVITY DIET

DANA WELLS

The mind of man is capable of anything.

— JOSEPH CONRAD

BRAIN FOOD DIET

CONTENTS

INTRODUCTION

Congratulations on purchasing *Brain Food Diet: Cognitive Decline and Alzheimer's Disease Reversed with Anti-aging Longevity Diet* and thank you for doing so. This book contains powerful, revolutionary information about how you can protect your brain and even help to undo some early signs of Alzheimer's disease just by changing your diet! Based on cutting-edge nutritional and neurological research, the dietary guidelines in this book have been proven to help keep your brain young and healthy for life.

You may be under the impression that there is nothing you can do to prevent your brain's inevitable decay and decline into memory loss, but that simply isn't true. While genetics can play a part in how likely you may be to develop Alzheimer's disease, there are many lifestyle changes that you can make to protect your brain. The most important change you can make is in the food you eat every day! Many people are unaware of how important diet can be in the fight against dementia and brain diseases like Alzheimer's. The following chapters will discuss all of the different foods you should include in your diet to optimize your brain's health.

Prepare yourself to learn many surprising truths about food that you cannot afford to live without. For example, you may be excited to learn how important fats and carbohydrates are for protecting your brain and preventing or even reversing the signs of brain decline. These may be foods that you have tried to eliminate from your diet because you thought they were bad for you, but in reality, they are an essential part of a brain-healthy diet. You will also discover what kinds of protein, as well as what sources of vitamins and minerals are key to improving your memory abilities and other cognitive functions. You may also be excited to discover that certain "treats" are powerful brain boosters!

Although this guide was written based on sound scientific research, it was not written by a doctor and should not be considered a substitute for medical advice. Always consult your health professional before making any changes to your diet, and be sure to seek a medical opinion if you have any concerns about your memory or other cognitive abilities. The author is not responsible for the outcome of following this or any other dietary advice.

There are many books on this subject on the market, so thanks again for choosing this one! Every effort was made to ensure that it is full of as much useful information as possible. Please enjoy!

PART I

UNDERSTANDING THE BRAIN AND NEURONUTRITION

1

TODAY'S BRAIN CRISIS

MUCH TO MY CHAGRIN, I MUST START THIS BOOK ON A SAD NOTE. WE are facing a crisis, and it does us no good to sugar-coat it or skirt around the truth. The number of people suffering from age-related cognitive decline, including Alzheimer's disease and other types of dementia, is steadily increasing. This disturbing truth has touched many of us as we have helplessly witnessed the decline of loved ones or have heard the pain in a friend's voice as they described the suffering of a beloved family member.

As strange as it may seem, this devastating increase of brain disorders in the elderly is, in part, due to the improvement of healthcare. The rapid advancement of medical care means that people are staying physically healthy for longer and are more likely to live well into their 70s, 80s, and even 90s. There are many examples of medical innovations that are helping people to live longer. For example, because of the success of current vaccinations against infectious diseases, fewer people die in their early years from fatal, contagious illnesses such as smallpox or measles. Additionally, people are also more likely to survive strokes and heart disease now than they were even just a decade ago.

Because people are avoiding killer childhood illnesses and surviving potentially fatal medical problems that can occur in young adults and middle-aged individuals, we are living longer, healthier lives. Unfortunately, this means that we are increasingly likely to survive to an age in which we are susceptible to Alzheimer's disease and other forms of dementia. The current greatest known risk factor for developing Alzheimer's disease is simply one's age. Although Alzheimer's disease is not necessarily a normal part of growing old, it is more likely to develop as we grow older.

What is Dementia and Alzheimer's Disease?

Before we go further into the investigation of what causes dementia and Alzheimer's disease, it is good to define a few terms. *Dementia* is something of a generic term that is used to describe a decrease in cognitive (mental) ability. To be classified as dementia, the mental decline must be severe enough to affect a person's lifestyle negatively.

Dementia classifies a group of symptoms including memory loss, decreased abilities in communication and language, reduced focus and ability to pay attention, lowered reasoning and judgment skills, and a decline in visual perception, which means making sense of what the eyes see. A person with dementia may only notice some of these symptoms, but they must show a noticeable decline in at least two areas for their condition to be considered dementia.

Although almost everyone occasionally has trouble remembering appointments or misplaces their keys from time to time, the symptoms of true dementia are significant enough to decrease a person's quality of life, and often, their ability to live independently. Most types of dementia are progressive, meaning that symptoms get worse over time, and some forms lead to fatal complications.

Some types of dementia are more well-known than others. There are a few kinds of dementia that are treatable and even reversible, usually because they are secondary to some other condition. Examples of reversible types of dementia include temporary dietary deficiencies (e.g., dangerously low vitamin B12), depression, alcoholism, temporary inflammation of the brain, and exposure to certain toxins in the environment.

Unfortunately, the most common forms of dementia are irreversible, although medications can sometimes slow the progression of symptoms. The second most common form of dementia is *vascular dementia*, which happens as a result of changes in the brain when a stroke occurs. In this form, mental abilities decline because blood flow to the brain is blocked. When less blood is flowing to the brain, its cells do not get adequate oxygen or other nutrients, and permanent damage can be done.

By sheer numbers, *Alzheimer's disease* is the most common form of dementia, accounting for some 60 to 80 percent of all dementia cases. Like many other forms of dementia, Alzheimer's symptoms get progressively worse over time. In the early stages of the disease, a person may experience only mild memory loss, but people in later stages of Alzheimer's may not be aware of their surroundings or be unable to communicate.

The Rise of Alzheimer's-Related Deaths

Currently, Alzheimer's disease is listed as the 6th leading cause of death in the United States. Although people cannot die directly from the disease, it is from complications caused by it that are ultimately fatal. In late stages, patients often lose weight and become very susceptible to fatal infections. They also have trouble with physical movements, including swallowing and inhaling food, which can lead to aspiration pneumonia. Additionally, because a complication like pneumonia may sometimes be listed on the death certificate, the actual number of people who have passed away from underlying Alzheimer's disease is not known. One study estimated that up to 500,000 people might have died from Alzheimer's in the United States in 2010 alone!

As mentioned earlier, death rates from dementia and Alzheimer's disease are currently rising. In the U.S., approximately 17.6 people per 100,000 died from Alzheimer's in 2000. In the year 2015, this number nearly doubled to 34.4 people per 100,000 and the numbers that show the ages of those affected by Alzheimer's are even more startling. In people ages 65 through 74, the number of people per 100,000 who died from Alzheimer's only rose slightly in those 15 years from 18.7 to 22.4 people. However, in people aged 85 or older, the number of people who died from the disease rose from 667.7 per 100,000 in 2000 to 1,174.2 per 100,000 people in 2015. Population predictions currently show that by 2050, there will be approximately 32 million people over the age of 80 in the United States, about half of whom will have Alzheimer's disease.

All of these statistics tell us that the number of people dying from Alzheimer's disease is increasing, especially among the very elderly. Although you may be relatively young right now and may not currently have anyone in your life who suffers from any form of dementia, this rise in people living with Alzheimer's has the potential to affect everyone. People who are 65 and older typically survive 4 to 8 years after being diagnosed with Alzheimer's, though some may live for up to 20 years with this disease. That is an incredibly long time to live with a disease that is extremely difficult to cope with, not only for the sufferer but also for their loved ones. It is unbelievably painful and frustrating to watch the slow mental decline of someone you love and to see their personality disappear before your eyes. It takes a tremendous toll on the patient, caregivers, families, friends, and the community around them.

The majority of people who die from dementia typically spend the last part of their lives in nursing homes. Among people who live in nursing homes, the number who have Alzheimer's is significantly higher than those who are suffering from other conditions, including cancer. Given that people can live for so many years with Alzheimer's disease and so many families have to move their loved ones into extended care facilities, the disease has a huge impact on public health concerning expenses and the overall allocation of resources. This statement is not meant to sound cold as dementia patients certainly deserve the very best of care, but if Alzheimer's were less prevalent, more medical resources could be used for treating and preventing other diseases, like cancer.

Alzheimer's and other forms of dementia are so widespread, and their impact on society is so great, that we can safely say these conditions have reached epidemic proportions. The cost of care for people with Alzheimer's and other forms of dementia in the United States during 2018 alone has been estimated at $277 billion. Note that this number does not include unpaid care such as that given by family members.

Currently, there is no scientifically known cure for Alzheimer's or other progressive forms of dementia. These are very complex diseases, so treatment typically focuses on slowing the rate of mental decline so that the patient can enjoy a certain quality of life for as long as possible. There are various drugs aimed at treating Alzheimer's symptoms, and they do help with some patients, however, these medications generally only help for a limited time. Ultimately, although these treatments may delay it for a time, they are unable to change the progressive nature of the disease.

So, What Causes Dementia or Alzheimer's Disease?

Strictly speaking, most dementia, including Alzheimer's disease, involves the continual wasting and eventual death of brain cells, which causes the symptoms of decreased mental ability. But what causes these brain cells to begin wasting away in the first place?

As it turns out, there is a complicated answer to this simple question. For a long time, Alzheimer's was thought to be a nearly unavoidable result of growing older, especially if one had the genetic predisposition to the disease. However, it turns out that the causes of Alzheimer's are much more complicated than this prior understanding. As the understanding of what causes Alzheimer's and many other forms of age-related dementia changes, we are beginning to see clues that there may be hope for better prevention of these conditions, and possibly even a cure.

Here's Where We Finally Hear the Good News

It is true that having a particular form of a specific gene *does* make a person more likely to develop Alzheimer's later in life, but it does not make the disease something that is inevitable. More and more, current research is leading scientists to understand that there are many other lifestyle factors including physical activity, the amount of stimulation a person's brain receives, and the types of food we eat that also influence our likelihood to develop age-related forms of dementia such as Alzheimer's disease. In short, your genes are not your fate. Recent research shows that less than one percent of those who have Alzheimer's disease have the type of gene that causes an increased risk of the disease. Everyone else who has Alzheimer's developed it as a result of other lifestyle-related factors.

This news should be met with resounding cheers because it means that we no longer need to live our lives in the anticipation that, if we are lucky enough to live into our 80s, we will face the foggy and painful decline associated with dementia. Instead of settling for that fatalistic mindset, it turns out that we can take steps toward keeping our brains healthy and preventing dementia *right now*!

As researchers uncover more information about how nutrition affects our brain health, they understand how the concept of *epigenetics* is associated with how quickly our brains decline with age. Simply put, epigenetics is how certain genes can be turned on and off by various life circumstances.

Epigenetics is a fairly new scientific field, and one of its primary focuses is our lifestyles, including the foods we choose to eat. In a nutshell, an important discovery of epigenetics is that although our genes may increase our chances of developing diseases such as Alzheimer's, our diets and physical activity levels also have great influence over whether or not we develop those diseases.

It's the classic nature vs. nurture debate all over again. So, although nature (in this case, our genetic make-up) has a lot of control over our physical makeup, it doesn't pre-determine everything about us. Countless characteristics of our appearances, personalities, and internal functions are also influenced by the environments in which we are raised (the *nurture* factor). As we become adults, the ways our genes are expressed continue to be influenced by the choices we make – you might say by the way we nurture ourselves.

Much of how we nurture ourselves has to do with our diets. Each day, we have the power to choose whether we eat healthy foods or not-so-healthy foods. While some of us are limited by finances and the availability of healthy foods, most of us do have some control over what we put in our bodies. Particularly in industrialized nations like the U.S., we face an overabundance of diet choices, but unfortunately, many of the most tempting choices are detrimental to the health of our bodies, especially our brains.

In the next couple of chapters, you will be introduced to the wonderful inner workings of your amazing brain and get a quick look at just how much influence your diet can have on your brain's health. Hold on tight – you're in for an exciting, educational, and often surprising journey!

INTRODUCING THE BRAIN

WHILE IT'S TRUE THAT ALL ANIMALS HAVE BRAINS, THE HUMAN BRAIN is truly special and unique in its form and function for a variety of reasons. For one thing, human beings have a superior ability to problem solve, be imaginative, and communicate in both written and oral forms in a complex way to which no other member of the animal kingdom compares. Among the many important jobs of the brain are the following: controlling your body's temperature, breathing, heart rate, and blood pressure; making sense of all that you see, hear, smell, touch, and taste; telling your body parts how and when to move; and allowing you to think, feel, and dream.

To help you fully appreciate this marvelous organ and to recognize just how critical it is for you to protect it via your diet, this chapter contains a little tour of the human brain. This overview will, by no means, be comprehensive, but it should be enough to give you a basic idea of its overall structure and function.

The Central and Peripheral Nervous System

Just as your stomach is part of the digestive system, your brain is also a part of the nervous system. Your nervous system consists of the *central nervous system*, which includes the brain and spinal cord, and the *peripheral nervous system*, which covers the rest of the nerves of the body. Together, these two parts of the nervous system work to control and regulate the workings of the entire body - talk about a big job!

Neurons – The Basic Unit of the Brain

The main cell type within the brain and the nervous system is called a *neuron*, and your brain has 100 billion of these little cells! Like other cells, they have the main body, which houses a nucleus, and other typical components that are found in most types of cells. Additionally, like most other types of cells, they have a very specific job. In the case of neurons, their job is to transmit messages from the brain to the body, and back from the body to the brain. These messages take the form of electric impulses, which travel from neuron to neuron until they have reached their destination at either a specific part of the brain or at a specific part of the body.

However, unlike other types of cells in the body, neurons have branches coming from the body called *dendrites* which receive messages that are sent from other neurons; these messages then travel into the cell body. Another extension of the cell body of a neuron is called an *axon*. This part is typically longer than dendrites, and its job is to carry messages away from the cell body.

The lengths of some axons are covered by a *myelin sheath*, which is made up of fatty material and acts as a sort of insulation that helps electrical signals stay strong along the entire length (without dissipating outwards into space outside of the axon). It also helps the message travel faster. Axons end in *axon terminals*, which pass the electrical impulse along to other neurons. In between two neurons is a gap called a *synapse*. In this gap, specific chemical interactions take place to transmit messages between neuron cells.

All of the messages that travel along the neurons between the body and brain can happen almost instantly! A good example is the last time you touched a hot stove and quickly withdrew your hand. For that to happen, your hand had to send a message to your brain about what it felt; then, your brain had to send a message back about how it (the hand) should react by quickly withdrawing. That's some super-fast messaging – even faster than high school kids can text message each other these days!

There are three main types of neurons, and they all have slightly different structures. The individual structures of each neuron type are not important for you to remember just now, as long as you remember the basic parts described below. The first neuron we will cover is *motor neurons* which carry messages from the brain and spinal cord (central nervous system) to the rest of your body, including your muscles and organs. The second are *sensory neurons* which do the opposite and carry messages from your body's various parts to the spinal cord and brain. The third type, *interneurons*, form connections between neurons within the central nervous system and carry messages between motor neurons and sensory neurons.

Brain Parts

The brain includes three main parts: the brain stem, the cerebellum, and the cerebrum.

The *brain stem* links your spinal cord to the brain and controls essential automatic functions such as your breathing and heart rate. It is also responsible for your reflexes, consciousness, and organ functions such as digestion. It also has important functions when it comes to your sleep.

Below and behind the main part of your brain is the *cerebellum* which is a small ball of tissue that receives important information from your muscles, eyes, and ears. It then uses this information to help coordinate the movements of your arms and legs.

The main part of the brain, the *cerebrum*, is the large part that many people think of as the entire brain. It's easy to forget about the other parts, but as you can tell from their descriptions, they are all indispensable! The cerebrum consists of many different parts and is divided in half into two hemispheres. As a whole, this part of the brain combines information from all of the sensory organs, controls your emotions, keeps track of your thoughts and memories, and is responsible for the initiation of all of your conscious movements.

The two *hemispheres* of your brain are the right and left sides. You have heard of people being "right-brained" if they have creative tendencies or "left-brained" if they have an orderly, logical personality. In truth, however, we all use both sides of our brains. The left hemisphere is in charge of your speech and language abilities, while the right hemisphere gives you important spatial information, like telling you where your foot happens to be right now.

Each hemisphere is divided into four lobes. The *frontal lobes* (where your forehead is) are in charge of thinking, problem-solving, movement, short-term memory, and organizing, whereas the *parietal lobes* (directly behind the frontal lobes) take information from your sensory organs and interpret it so that you know what you are tasting, touching, hearing, and seeing. Further, the *occipital lobes* (at the back of your head) take images from your eyes and process them to link them with images that your memory has stored. Finally, the *temporal lobes* process information from the senses of hearing, smell, and taste; they also assist with memory storage.

One extremely noteworthy area of the brain called the *limbic system* is located deep within the cerebrum, tucked away by the top of the brain stem. The structures in this part control memories and emotions, and it consists of the thalamus, hypothalamus, and hippocampus. The *hippocampus* helps control the storage of memories, sending them to the correct sections of the cerebrum and then recalling them later. The *thalamus* receives the motor and sensory signals from the body, then relays them to the cerebrum. The *hypothalamus* controls your emotions, regulates your body's temperature, and controls important urges, such as those to sleep and eat.

The Blood-Brain Barrier

One of the most fascinating and essential parts of brain function is the *blood-brain barrier*. Like all other organs, the brain relies on an intricate network of blood vessels to bring oxygen and nutrient-rich blood to its cells, and to carry blood away once it has been depleted of oxygen and important nutrients. However, unlike other organs, the brain has a security system known as the blood-brain barrier.

For the environment of the brain to remain stable enough to constantly and consistently transmit messages, it is critical that only specific essential materials are allowed in and out of the blood that bathes this organ. This network of blood vessels surrounding the brain lets important nutrients in while protecting against potentially harmful foreign substances.

Unlike vessels around other organs, the blood vessels around the brain are lined with cells that are so tightly wedged together that they are nearly impossible to penetrate. This protection keeps bacteria, toxins, and all other unwanted substances from entering the brain. However, the brain does depend on receiving important nutrients, along with hormones, that are sent from the body's other organs.

Through decades of study, researchers have discovered more about how the blood-brain barrier allows important molecules to pass through. Essentially, anything that is very small or *fat-soluble* (able to be dissolved in fat) can slip out of the brain's blood vessels. This easy passage allows many hormones, anti-depressants, and anti-anxiety medications to enter the brain. Unfortunately, many harmful chemicals like alcohol and cocaine can also gain entry to the brain in this way.

Large molecules that are needed by the brain, like insulin, glucose, and amino acids, are taken across the barrier by *transporter proteins* which are located in the lining of the brain's blood vessels. These proteins are specific to the type of molecule that they take across the barrier. For example, glucose transporter proteins only grab and pull glucose molecules across the wall while insulin must be taken across by a different type of transporter protein.

Research has shown that some neurodegenerative diseases might occur when the blood-brain barrier is weakened, it thus allows certain types of molecules across that it normally wouldn't allow. One example is multiple sclerosis (MS) where it is possible that a leaky barrier allows too many white blood cells into the brain. These white blood cells attack the myelin sheaths that line the axons, either slowing the electrical impulses or allowing them to dissipate so that they aren't sent at all. The degeneration of myelin leads to MS's many debilitating neurological symptoms.

One downside to the brain's sophisticated blood-brain barrier is that it does not allow potentially helpful drugs into the brain. Scientists and doctors are constantly working to find ways to "trick" this barrier so that lifesaving drugs can gain targeted access to different parts of the brain. Through this research, they hope to develop more treatments for brain tumors and neurodegenerative diseases like MS.

The Brain's Protection

The brain is also unique among the body's organs in that it is the very best protected part of the body. Each of us has a built-in helmet known as the *skull*. Eight bones surround the brain, and they are connected tightly to each other by immovable joints. Additional bones of the skull also protect your face – 14 bones, to be exact. The skull acts as armor and is very effective at shielding the brain from quite a lot of trauma.

Under the skull is an additional layer of protection. There are three layers of tissue called the *meninges*, which serve as a barrier between the brain and skull. A final protective layer is provided by *cerebrospinal fluid (CFS)*, which the brain and spinal cord float within. This fluid also helps cushion it and keep the unique shape of these precious organs. This triple layer of protection provides evidence of just how valuable the brain is to our bodies.

Evolution of the Human Brain

In the animal world, larger bodies generally house larger brains. A notable exception to this rule is seen in human brains, which, when compared to those of other primates and their evolutionary ancestors, are extremely complex and large. Even gorillas, whose bodies are quite massive, have smaller brains and far fewer neurons than humans. Researchers have been investigating the development and evolution of the human brain for decades, and the reason for our complex, large brain (when compared to our relatively puny non-gorilla bodies) seems to boil down to the nutrition our ancestors ate.

The sheer complexity and vast abilities of our human brains require a calorically dense diet. Our brains consume about 20 percent of our body's energy when we are resting. This means that the appetite of our brains is twice the relative energy requirements of other primate brains, which take a mere 10 percent of their resting energy needs. Fortunately, we humans have the advantage of being able to consume and digest meat, which tends to contain far more energy than plants. It has been estimated that for a gorilla to feed a humanlike brain, it would need more than 700 additional calories each day. Since gorillas are vegetarians and already spend about 10 hours eating per day, supplying this much additional nutrition would be almost impossible.

On top of eating meat, humans can cook food, making more foods accessible for consumption throughout the year. The process of cooking also makes more nutrients digestible from all kinds of food, both vegetables, and meats. The ability to cook is clearly an additional advantage that humans have over our modern primate counterparts.

Evolutionary researchers and archaeologists who look specifically at skull sizes of human ancestors have come up with scientifically supported estimates of their brain sizes. They noted a dramatic growth spurt in brains approximately 800,000 years ago, ultimately leading to humans being nearly fully evolved with large brains close to today's sizes about 250,000 years ago. Their well-researched theories suggest that, at some point around the growth spurt, humans must have begun preparing food by cooking it, including meat in their diets, or a combination of both of these advantages.

These nutritional advantages were the only ways that early humans could have supported the demands of their increasingly large and complex brains. If they had stuck to a raw, plant-based diet, their hungry brains would have required them to spend their entire days foraging and eating, which would not have been conducive to avoiding predation.

The evolutionary link between nutrition and the development of modern human brains provides a valuable clue as to how our diets can continue to shape our brains throughout our lifetimes. We'll look into this concept further in the next chapter as we prepare to dive into the world of brain nutrition.

3

YOU ARE WHAT YOU EAT

THE MORE SCIENTISTS LOOK INTO THE EFFECT THAT NUTRITION HAS on our bodies, the more they realize that we are what we eat. In the field of neurological studies, current research is revealing just how impactful our diet is on the health of our brains. These studies have become so important that they have birthed an entirely new field called *neuro-nutrition*.

Neuro-nutrition

Neuro-nutrition is also known as "nutritional cognitive neuroscience" by some. This new scientific field combines neurology and nutrition to look into the effects of the foods we eat on brain health and cognitive powers over a lifespan.

Although humans have been interested in using food and nutrients to improve health and treat or prevent diseases for a millennium, the demand for answers to the Alzheimer's and dementia crisis has forced nutritional researchers to focus more specifically on the brain recently. This demand has come about because, thus far, modern medicine has not come up with a way to cure or prevent these and other devastating brain diseases with drugs or other medical treatments.

This new research has revealed that nutrition plays a tremendously important role in how well our brains work and how they age. Some foods have now been classified as "*neuroprotective*," meaning that they help to defend the brain from harm, and support its health regardless of a person's stage of life. However, some foods have an adverse effect and can cause real harm to the brain, thereby increasing your risk of dementia down the road. In fact, despite the unique defense of the blood-brain barrier, the brain is more easily damaged by a harmful diet than any other organ in the body. More than most other organs, the brain depends on a regular influx of necessary nutrients to keep it running at peak performance. If we consistently fail to give our brains what they need, a lifetime of nutritional deficits can cause this organ to age and fail much more quickly than it would if we had given it the proper nutrients.

Nutrigenetics

Scientists have gone even further into this research with the realization that no two people are exactly alike regarding their nutritional requirements for optimal health. We are all made up of a unique set of genes within our DNA, and as a result, our nutritional needs can vary greatly.

Remember the description of epigenetics in Chapter 1 as the study of how certain genes can be "switched on or off" by conditions in our environment? Well, the field of *nutrigenetics* delves even further into this field by specifically looking at how nutrition affects how our genetic traits are expressed. An obvious example of this is in people who have celiac disease, which is characterized by an extreme allergy to gluten. For example, if people with this disorder eat food products containing the protein gluten, their small intestines suffer severe damage from an attack by their immune systems. The solution, of course, is to avoid foods containing gluten at all costs, which is sometimes a deed that is easier said than done. Since celiac disease is linked to a genetic predisposition, this is an example of how following nutritional guidelines based on our unique genetics can alter how our DNA expresses itself.

Another example of nutrigenetics in action can be seen in the particular form of one gene that makes individuals more likely to develop Alzheimer's disease later in life. If someone with this form of the gene were to eat foods that are proven to be neuroprotective throughout their lifetime while also avoiding foods that are harmful to the brain, they would most likely have a significantly reduced chance of developing any form of dementia later in life, regardless of what their DNA says.

In contrast, many people who do not have the so-called "Alzheimer's gene" are *not* eating the right kinds of food for optimal brain health. These people, whether they are aware of it or not, are putting themselves at extreme risk of significant cognitive decline and possible dementia when they reach their 80s, 70s, or even 60s, even if they don't have the genetic predisposition for Alzheimer's disease.

So, how have researchers come to discover which foods are brain-healthy? Well, countless studies have helped scientists discover and confirm this information. By studying brain structure and function, and coming to understand the types of molecules that are critical to this organ's processes, neurologists now know exactly which vitamins, minerals, hormones, proteins, and other nutrients are required to keep the brain running smoothly. Conversely, they have also been able to observe and identify which nutrients wreak havoc on brain function when ingested. By identifying foods that contain these brain-healthy and brain-harmful nutrients, researchers have been able to come up with more specific recommendations regarding how to eat for optimal brain health.

Additionally, key research in neuro-nutrition has centered around studying populations that have a high percentage of seniors who are in good health, both mentally and physically. By looking at the lifestyles of these healthy elders, specifically by looking at their diets, neuroscientists began to get an understanding of the kinds of diets that are most supportive of brain health and dementia prevention.

Specifically, researchers have focused on people who live to be 100 years or older who have been described using the term "centenarians." Scientists who specifically research various aspects of aging have spent a considerable amount of time and effort looking at populations in parts of the world with the greatest concentrations of centenarians. Their goal has been and continues to be the determination of the characteristics of these populations that contribute to such healthy longevity in their citizens. As a result of these studies, many factors have been discovered that contribute to healthy aging, including positive outlooks on life, lower stress rates, strong social and family networks, avoiding smoking, physical activity, small body size, and diet.

Some areas with the greatest concentrations of centenarians are located on the Japanese island of Okinawa, in the European country of Bulgaria, on the Nicoya Peninsula of Costa Rica, on the Greek island of Ikaria, and on the island of Sardinia, Italy. The only comparative population in the United States is located in Loma Linda, California, where the population is primarily made up of people belonging to the Seventh-Day Adventist Church. By looking at the diets of these and other populations with high concentrations of the "oldest-old", researchers have come up with a comprehensive list of dietary recommendations to keep our brains healthy for a lifetime. These recommendations are relevant to everyone, since, as previously mentioned, people are living longer and longer these days. In other words, if we're most likely going to live a long life, we might as well keep our brains healthy while we're at it. Wouldn't it be nice to reach our 80s with a memory and other cognitive powers that are still fully intact?

Although there are many cultural and regional differences between each of those places with high populations of centenarians, their diets have a few key characteristics in common. These populations generally avoid processed foods in favor of whole, nutrient dense foods that they prepare themselves. They also eat very little meat, concentrating instead on a mainly plant-based diet including nuts, beans, whole grains, vegetables, and fruits. Additionally, any meat that they do eat comes from organic, pasture-raised, or free-range sources which do not include unnatural antibiotics, hormones, or any other foreign toxin or chemicals. Many of these populations also include a lot of healthy fish in their diets.

It should be noted that these populations also have a few other important attributes in common aside from healthy diets. In general, they emphasize family and community values, with strong moral principles and respect for each other. Additionally, elders are held in high esteem, and many of them work or remain physically active for nearly their entire lives, yet another factor that helps keep the brain and body healthy for a lifetime. However, they have also managed to accomplish balance in their lives, meaning that they take time for leisurely social activities and for resting and recharging their bodies.

These characteristics are all things that we would do well to incorporate into our lives in the United States where we typically overemphasize work for the first part of our lives, exhausting ourselves and staying extremely busy, only to come to a screeching halt, both physically and mentally, once we reach our 60s or 70s. This pattern seems to represent the exact opposite of the lifestyle of healthy centenarians. As a whole, the culture in the U.S. lacks a healthy sense of balance between work and play.

In the next section, we'll briefly look at a couple of brain-healthy diets that have gained popularity in recent years. Then, in Part 2 of this guide, we'll break down all the healthy nutrients that are needed by the brain. As you'll learn, the previously-described populations have the right idea when it comes to eating for long-term brain health!

Brain-Healthy Diets

These days, we read about countless fad diets that claim to be the latest solution to all of our health problems and it's hard to know whom to trust. For example, if you want to lose weight, should you follow the keto diet or the Atkins diet, right? To "detoxify" your body, is Whole30 the right plan for you or should you try switching to the Paleo diet? Should you go gluten-free for optimal health? The options are mind-boggling, and you cannot always be sure whether the guidelines for such diets are based on real research or if they're just based on pseudo-science that makes unfounded claims.

Although this book is not a comprehensive guide to nutrition for all parts of your body, it can certainly ease your mind about which diets are grounded in science among the ones that best serve your brain health. An added benefit of these diets is that, in general, the foods that best serve your brain are also good for your cardiovascular function (your heart and lungs) as well as the rest of your body. Here is a brief breakdown of these brain-healthy diets:

The Mediterranean Diet

It's no wonder that two of the densest populations of centenarians reside in Italy and Greece. One of the best diets for your brain is one that mimics the recipes and traditional foods of Mediterranean cooking. This diet was originally popularized for its benefits to our hearts because of its association with healthy cholesterol levels. However, it turns out that the nutrition that is good for your heart is also great for your brain! Although modern commercially packaged foods have infiltrated the entire industrialized world, the principles and main foods of this diet can still be found in many parts of the countries around the Mediterranean Sea, especially on islands and along coastlines.

Here are the main principles of the Mediterranean diet:

- **Eat a lot of fruits and vegetables.** On the Mediterranean diet, you should aim to eat 7 to 10 servings of these so that plants make up the majority of your diet. Don't limit yourself to just a few fruits or veggies —experiment, mix it up, and try a variety! Many of these foods contain vast quantities of antioxidants and fiber, along with other necessary vitamins and minerals. Additionally, fruit helps healthily satisfy your sugar cravings.
- **Switch to olive oil or canola oil.** Instead of using butter as a cooking base, use these oils for sautéing and grilling, and try using flavored olive oil as a dip or spread for your bread.
- **Eat whole grains.** Any bread or grain product(s) you eat should be made only with whole grains. Avoid refined flours that you find in white bread and many kinds of

pasta. Instead, choose whole oats and brown rice over their more processed counterparts.

- **Eat more fish.** Unless you already eat a lot of fish, try to up your intake to once or twice a week. The best choices are fatty fish that have a high concentration of omega-3 fatty acids, like fresh or canned tuna, herring, salmon, trout, and mackerel. Prepare it by poaching, grilling, or sautéing in a little olive oil or canola oil, baking it, or broiling it. Obviously, it's best to avoid fried fish. Additionally, you should limit your intake of larger fish that are high in mercury, such as large tuna, certain mackerel, and sea bass, to only a couple times per month.

- **Limit your red meat intake.** Get the majority of your protein from vegetable sources, fish, and poultry. When you do eat red meat, make sure that it is lean and limit the portion size to about 3 ounces.

- **Use herbs and spices.** Add flavor and cut out unnecessary salt.

- **Snack on nuts.** A handful of nuts makes a good quick snack. Other good choices are all-natural peanut butter or tahini (a spread made from sesame seeds) as a dip for veggies.

- **Eat low-fat dairy products.** Switch from whole or 2 percent milk, yogurt, and cheese to their skim or low-fat counterparts.

- **Drink red wine sparingly.** A glass of red wine has health benefits, but don't go overboard as too much alcohol is harmful to your brain and the rest of your body. If you don't drink or shouldn't drink alcohol, there is no reason to start.

- **Hydrate!** Your main beverage while on this diet should be water. Coffee and tea are okay, but avoid any beverage that is sweetened with sugar or artificial sweeteners.

Besides what you eat, the Mediterranean lifestyle emphasizes a few other healthy practices, like enjoying meals with other people, savoring every bite, and getting plenty of physical activity each day.

This diet is rich in brain health benefits, and you'll get explanations of the specifics as you get into the second part of this book.

The DASH Diet

The name of this diet stands for "Dietary Approaches to Stop Hypertension". Hypertension is the same as high blood pressure, so this diet was created with the goal of lowering blood pressure in individuals for whom this is a problem. This diet was publicized after years of intensive research in the 1990s, primarily conducted by the U.S. National Institutes of Health (NIH). These studies showed that following the principles of this diet can help to lower high blood pressure, especially when combined with regular physical exercise. Lower blood pressure leads to a reduced risk of heart disease in many individuals.

Although it was not created to boost brain health, incidental side benefits that some DASH dieters and researchers have noticed is improved mental abilities. If you compare it to the other diets listed here and the descriptions of nutrients in the second part of this book, you'll see that it contains many components of a neuroprotective diet. Additional research has also suggested that the DASH diet may lead to a decreased risk of certain cancers, metabolic syndrome, and diabetes. For these reasons, the DASH diet is certainly worth consideration as a long-term healthy diet.

Instead of listing certain foods to eat, the DASH diet recommends specific servings within each food groups. These can be adjusted based on how many calories you need to consume to maintain a healthy weight. Be sure to discuss your daily calorie requirements with your doctor, and adjust the number of servings you eat according to his or her recommendations. Here is a general outline of the DASH diet's guidelines adjusted for 2,000 calories a day:

Dairy – 2 to 3 servings a day. These should be low fat or fat-free, just as in the Mediterranean diet. One principle of the DASH diet is low sodium intake, so be careful with cheeses, as they can be very high in sodium. Some examples of serving sizes are:

- 1.5 ounces of part-skim cheese
- 1 cup of skim or low-fat milk
- 1 cup of low-fat or fat-free yogurt
- 1/2 cup of low-fat cottage cheese

Lean meat, fish, and poultry – 6 or fewer servings a day. This amount sounds like a lot, but the serving sizes are quite small. Red meat should be eaten no more than twice a week or less, and be sure to pick leaner cuts. Serving sizes are:

- 1 egg, cooked as desired (as long as you follow the DASH recommendations for cooking oils, described later)
- 1 ounce of cooked lean meat, poultry, or fish

Whole Grains – 6 to 8 servings a day. Similar to the Mediterranean diet, avoid refined grains since they lack fiber and nutrients. Some whole grains are brown rice, 100% whole wheat bread, 100% whole wheat pasta, oatmeal, quinoa, and whole grain breakfast cereals (look for those with lower sugar, though). Typical serving sizes would be:

- ½ cup of cooked cereal, whole wheat pasta, oats, or rice

- 1 slice of bread
- 1 ounce of whole grain breakfast cereal

Fruits – 4 to 5 servings a day. These make for a healthy snack, usually require little to no prep, and are typically loaded with fiber. They are also versatile and can easily become a healthy dessert or a sweet addition to any salad. Serving sizes look like:

- A medium piece of fruit
- 4 ounces of fruit juice (beware of added sugars, though)
- ¼ cup of dried fruit (again, without added sugar)
- ½ cup of canned, frozen, or fresh fruits (make sure that any canned fruit is packed in light syrup, juice, or water instead of heavy syrup)

Veggies – 4 to 5 servings a day. There are no restrictions for which types of vegetables you can eat because all are acceptable with this diet. They can be used in many dishes and often substituted for some of the meat in certain recipes. If you use canned vegetables or frozen vegetables, look for the ones that have reduced sodium or are labeled as "no added salt." Servings might look like:

- ½ cup sliced or chopped, raw or cooked vegetables (this includes previously frozen or canned veggies)
- 1 cup of raw, leafy green veggies (like spinach, kale, lettuce, or bok choy)

Oils and Fats – 2 to 3 servings a day. Choose vegetable oils over those derived from animals. In other words, nix the butter and lard for olive, safflower, and canola oil. Soft margarine, light salad dressing, and low-fat mayo are also acceptable. Typical servings are:

- 2 tbsp light dressing or 1 tbsp of mayo
- 1 tsp soft margarine
- 1 tsp veggie oil, like olive or canola oil

Legumes, Nuts, and Seeds – 4 to 5 servings a week. Be sure you read that carefully – that's servings per week, not per day! Examples of these types of foods are canned and dried beans, lentils, almonds, cashews, peanuts, nut butter, peas, and flaxseeds. These have a lot of protein, fiber, and essential minerals. Serving sizes would look like:

- ½ cup cooked peas or beans
- 2 tbsp of seeds or nut butter
- 1/3 cup (a handful) of nuts

Sweet treats or added sugar – 5 or fewer servings a week. Eat candy very sparingly, and it's best to avoid soda altogether since it is hard to measure the amount of sugar you consume in these. Keep in mind that just one tablespoon of sugar contains 12.5 grams of sugar, which is a whole serving! Honey and agave nectar should also be restricted. Here are what sweet servings look like:

- ½ cup of sorbet
- 1 tbsp jelly, jam, or table sugar
- 1 cup of lemonade

Reduce your sodium intake. There are two variations to the DASH diet. On the *standard DASH diet*, you must limit yourself to 2,300 mg of sodium each day, and on the *lower sodium DASH diet*, the limit is 1,500 mg of sodium each day. Be sure to study nutrition labels before buying or consuming anything. It is shocking to learn how much salt goes into many prepackaged foods! Talk to your doctor about how much sodium you should be getting before choosing one of these plans. To boost flavor, experiment with different herbs, spices, or sodium-free salt substitutes.

Limit caffeine and alcohol. Although the DASH diet does not specifically address these, caffeine can temporarily increase your blood pressure, so limit yourself to the equivalent of 1 to 2 cups of coffee each day. Additionally, be sure to stick to the healthy recommendation of no more than 2 alcoholic drinks per day for men or 1 alcoholic drink per day for women.

The benefits of the DASH diet are more noticeable with regular physical exercise, so be sure to include physical activity in your daily life along with these dietary changes.

The MIND Diet

If you are torn between the two diets you just read about, here's some great news – there is a hybrid of the two called the MIND diet! This diet is very new, as it was just publicized in 2015. The MIND acronym stands for "Mediterranean-DASH Intervention for Neurodegenerative Delay." It was developed when researchers noticed that, although both of the diets in question had been shown to boost mental abilities, neither was created with the goal of specifically improving brain health or preventing the development of dementia. A team created this diet based on the neuroprotective qualities of both diets. Studies have proven that this plan is better for preventing age-related brain decay than either of the other two by themselves. One study showed that the risk of Alzheimer's disease was lowered by more than half by people who stuck to the diet very closely and by about a third by those who followed the diet a little more loosely.

Although it was created specifically for brain health, the MIND diet has recently been proven effective for weight loss, blood sugar control for diabetics, and improving heart health. Like the

Mediterranean and DASH diets, the MIND diet has recommendations for how many servings of various, healthy food groups you should eat as well as which foods you should avoid. Here is the breakdown:

- **Use olive oil.** Use this instead of any other oil or fat for cooking and flavor.
- **Eat fish a couple times a week if not more.** The best choices are those high in omega-3s, as outlined in the Mediterranean diet. Again, restrict your intake of fish that are high in mercury.
- **Include chicken or turkey.** These lean sources of protein should be included in your menu **at least twice a week.** Choose healthy preparation methods, like grilling or baking, instead of frying.
- **Berries are best.** Instead of indiscriminate consumption of all fruits, the MIND diet specifically recommends berries for their antioxidant levels. The plan suggests incorporating blueberries, strawberries, blackberries, and raspberries **at least two times per week.**
- **Eat your greens.** A serving of green leafy vegetables, such as kale, spinach, swiss chard, or romaine lettuce should be eaten **at least six times per week.**
- **Include other veggies, too.** A serving of another type of vegetable should be eaten **at least once per day.** Try to avoid those high in starch, like white potatoes and corn.
- **Don't forget the beans.** Add a serving of beans to your menu **four or more times each week.** Examples include black beans, kidney beans, lentils, soybeans, and garbanzo beans, also known as chickpeas.
- **Go nuts.** Incorporate a variety of different nuts into your diet, with **five or more servings per week.** Different types

of nuts contain different nutrients, so try to include a little of them all.

- **Eat a lot of whole grains.** Whole grains may be the most plentiful food group in this plan, with a recommended **three or more servings a day.** See the Mediterranean and DASH diets above for examples of whole grain types and servings.
- **Raise a glass of red wine.** That's it, just a glass. This would be 3 ounces for a woman and 5 ounces for a man.

The MIND diet also lists a few specific foods to avoid or limit for better brain health primarily because they contain saturated or trans fats. These recommendations are as follows:

- **Less than four servings of red meat each week.** When you do eat red meat, aim for the leaner, less processed choices. In this case, "red meat" includes all pork, lamb, and beef.
- **Little or no fried food.** If you must eat something fried, do so **less than once a week.**
- **Very little cheese.** The MIND diet recommends **less than one serving each week.**
- **Limit butter and margarine to a tablespoon or less per day.** As stated above, use olive oil for cooking or for dipping bread.
- **Watch your junk food intake.** By "junk food", the diet means ice cream, cookies, donuts, candy, and all other processed desserts or snacks. These are allowed **four times each week or less.**

Each of the diets listed has specific health benefits, but they have all been proven to boost brain health. If you choose to follow one, be sure to talk to your doctor first. If you are curious about other diets that have become popular in recent years and are wishing to reduce your risk of developing dementia, evaluate them based on the recommendations in Parts 2 and 3 of this book as they break down nutrients that are necessary for brain health as well as foods that can be harmful to the brain. Again, if you are interested in a specific diet, be sure to consider whether it follows the guidelines for better brain health!

4

HOW TO READ THIS BOOK

YOU SHOULD READ THIS BOOK AS AN EDUCATIONAL GUIDE FOR EATING with the specific goal of protecting your brain health. This book is not a weight-loss plan, although following these healthy recommendations may lead to some weight loss, especially if it is vastly different from how you have been eating.

The research and recommendations in this book should, by no means, be seen as a substitute for the advice of a health professional. Before making any dietary or exercise changes, you should always consult with your doctor. Be sure to undergo any necessary tests that he or she may recommend before you start a new diet.

Although the guidelines in this book are based on many years of research and careful study, results can and will vary among individuals.

The next two parts provide a breakdown of the critical nutrients that your brain needs for optimal health, as well as an explanation of the foods that can harm your cognitive powers. At times, specific serving sizes and servings per day may be recommended, but these may not always be included. Suggestions for food combinations will also be given, but ultimately, this is not a recipe book. Menu plans and recipes for the MIND, DASH, and Mediterranean diets are widely available from many popular sources. I highly recommend searching for these recipes or using what you have learned from this book to evaluate any other recipes that you may come across. You can also use the suggestions in this book to make brain-healthy substitutions, such as using olive oil instead of butter or quinoa instead of white rice.

PART II

BRAIN SUPERFOODS

5

WONDERFUL WATER

HAVE YOU EVER BEEN DEHYDRATED? WHEN YOU HEAR THE WORD "dehydrated," you probably think of a situation in which a person has collapsed from heat exhaustion and needs immediate IV fluids. However, the state of being dehydrated does not need to be anywhere nearly as dramatic as that type of situation. In fact, the reality is that most of us regularly experience some level of dehydration, even if it's just to a mild extent.

Every time you feel thirsty, it is a sign from your body that you are already somewhat dehydrated. Thirst is your body's way of communicating its need for hydration before a dire emergency takes place.

Time and again, you have heard doctors and nutrition experts recommend that you drink 8 to 10 glasses of water per day, but how many of us follow that recommendation? We may virtuously make an effort from time to time, but all too often distractions and business keep us from the essential task of hydrating our bodies.

Why is Water Important?

The reason that water is essential to all aspects of your health is that an adult human body contains approximately 11 gallons of water, give or take a bit depending on the size of the person. Additionally, your blood is made up of about 85% water, your muscles are 80% water, and your brain is 75% water.

On top of the sheer volume of water in your body is the fact that you are constantly losing water. Every time you exhale, a little water leaves your body in the form of vapor, hence why you can "fog up" a mirror or window when you breathe on it. When you sweat, even a little, water is lost. Even though your kidneys are very good at conserving water, you lose water from your body every time you urinate. All of this water must be replenished somehow, or every part of your body suffers!

This is Your Brain on Dehydration

Since your brain is mostly water, it shrinks when you are dehydrated. It contracts away from the skull, causing a common pain known as a "dehydration headache". This type of headache can be mild or quite severe. For example, if you've ever woken up with a hangover, much of the pain you experienced was the result of alcohol's dehydrating effects.

Beyond the physical pain of dehydration, your brain suffers other effects when you are not taking in enough fluid. Decades of research has shown that dehydration can lead to mental effects such as sleepiness, depressed mood or other mood impairment, and mental "fog", or confusion. In cognitive performance assessments, young children and older adults showed a decreased ability to think rationally when they were dehydrated. Healthy young adults were less dramatically affected, but even this population experiences memory problems and a reduction of other cognitive functions when their fluids are low. Another surprising effect that dehydration has on our nervous system is that it increases our sensitivity to pain.

How to Hydrate

The solution, of course, is to drink water and lots of it! Experts truly know what they are talking about when they recommend 8 to 10 glasses of water every day, and seniors should drink even more as they can typically become dehydrated more easily.

Plain water is all that is necessary to keep your brain running at peak hydration, and in advanced countries, we are fortunate to have access to abundant water. So, all you need to do is develop the habit of sipping on water throughout your day.

It is not even necessary to go out and buy a bunch of bottled water, though you may do so if that is your preference. Some experts claim that spring or mineral water contains more of the essential electrolytes and minerals that your body and brain require, while purified water lacks these essential nutrients. However, *any* water is better than no water at all! Sparkling water even works because it is simply water that has been "dressed up" with bubbles.

If you'd rather stick to plain tap water, consider investing in either a filter that attaches to your faucet or a water pitcher that contains a filter for tap water. Although your city's water is routinely tested for safety, sometimes things go awry, as evidenced by the recent lead crisis in Flint, Michigan. Filters also eliminate the taste and odor of chlorine, which is added to our water to kill harmful pathogens. This additive is necessary, but there is no need for us to ingest it!

Additionally, sometimes tap water contains trace levels of "safe" metals like zinc, iron, copper, and aluminum. These metals are considered essential nutrients for the human body because we need them in minute amounts. However, only tiny amounts of them are needed. Many studies have linked over-consumption of zinc, iron, copper, and aluminum with a possible increased risk of developing dementia. Since we get plenty of each of these elements in our food, it's best to play it safe and filter them out of our drinking water.

Other Hydration Sources

You may be wondering about other beverages and their ability to hydrate. Electrolyte-infused sports drinks can be useful, but these are only truly necessary when you have been working hard and sweating profusely. When you do drink them, look for ones with reduced sugar because, as you'll learn later, too much sugar does not do your brain any favors!

With that same idea in mind, think about sodas. While these do have the power to contribute to your hydration to a certain extent, when we drink them, our bodies have to process a lot of sugar, as well as other ingredients, which reduces their hydrating effects. Even artificial sweeteners keep diet sodas from being as hydrating as plain water. Coffee and tea follow a similar principle – even if they are unsweetened, the caffeine in them lowers their ability to hydrate you. However, they do contribute to your fluid levels somewhat, so don't count them out completely. Conversely, milk is a good source of hydration since it is about 90% water and does not contain any caffeine or too much sugar. The only beverages that are truly dehydrating are alcoholic beverages, so if you do choose to drink alcohol, be sure to drink a glass of water for each serving of alcohol unless you want to suffer the pain of a hangover in the morning.

All of the above beverages can help to contribute to your overall hydration to a certain extent. However, as you've undoubtedly learned from other sources, it's best for your health to limit your intake of sodas and other caffeinated beverages. So, your best bet for hydration is still plain water. If you find yourself bored and uninspired by plain old water, you can always dress it up a bit with a handful of berries, a few slices of citrus fruits, or even a sprig of mint or basil. These fruit and herb infusions add flavor without taking away from water's hydrating effects.

You can also get some of your hydration from fruits and vegetables. Although the water content of these varies, they can certainly contribute to your overall water intake. Some of the most hydrating fruits are in the melon family, such as watermelon, cantaloupe, and honeydew; citrus fruits like oranges and grapefruits also have high water content. Veggies that contain a lot of water include cucumbers, tomatoes, bell peppers, romaine lettuce, and celery.

How Can You Tell if You are Hydrated?

You may be wondering if there is any way to determine whether you are taking in enough fluids, and the key is to monitor your urinary output. If you urinate every 2 to 4 hours, the color of your urine is clear to light yellow, and there is a good volume of urine each time, you are probably taking in enough fluid. However, if you are not drinking enough, you will likely only urinate small amounts infrequently, and the color will vary from dark yellow to orange. This color is a sign that you should drink more water, pronto!

Other signs of dehydration are the aforementioned mental confusion and moodiness, dizziness, dry mouth, skin that does not bounce back quickly when you pinch it, reduced sweat output, increased pulse, and fatigue. If you experience these symptoms, severe dehydration may be impending or may have already arrived. You need to drink some water immediately. Cool water may be harder on the stomach, but it has been shown to absorb more quickly into the system than warmer water.

If symptoms of dehydration do not improve within 20 minutes of drinking a couple of glasses of water, it's best to seek medical help. Severe symptoms of dehydration include fever, delirium, loss of consciousness, and sunken eyes. In the case of any of these symptoms, medical intervention is required to replace intravenous fluids and salts. The best advice for preventing this from happening is to drink up, not only for your body but for the best brain health!

6

POWERFUL PROTEIN

THE BRAIN CONSISTS MAINLY OF FAT AND WATER, SO IT MAY SURPRISE you to learn that protein is an essential nutrient for peak cognitive function. You undoubtedly know that the rest of your body needs protein, as it is the building block for many different parts, including your hair, nails, bones, muscles, skin, and blood. Damaged tissue needs protein for repairs. Additionally, taking in enough protein is critical for healthy brain function and reducing your risk of developing dementia!

The Role of Protein in Your Body

Protein is essential to healthy brain function because it plays a central role in all of the processes that take place within this precious organ. Your brain relies on chemical reactions and chemical messengers for transmitting thoughts and impulses, initiating changes within your body, storing and retrieving memories, controlling your moods, and pretty much every single process that is controlled by the brain. The messengers and other molecules that take part in the brain's chemical reactions are made up of *amino acids*, which come from protein.

When you consume a source of protein, it is broken down by the digestive process into amino acids. The body then takes these amino acids and uses them to make new proteins and other molecules which serve in various important functions all over the body, including the brain. There are 21 amino acids that the body uses to make all of the proteins that it needs. Some sources will tell you that the body uses 20 amino acids, but the 21st one was found fairly recently, so those sources just haven't caught up to the most recent research.

Types of Amino Acids

Of those 21 amino acids, 9 of them are considered "*essential*" because your body cannot make them. Thus, you have to get them from the foods that you eat. If a food contains all 9 of these essential amino acids, it is considered a *complete protein source*. Many foods supply some, but not all of these amino acids, and are thus referred to as *incomplete protein sources.* However, these incomplete protein sources can be combined to form a complete protein source, so there are many options available for getting the protein you need. We'll get into the foods that supply these amino acids in just a little while.

Besides the 9 essential amino acids, the other 12 are considered either "*nonessential*" or "*conditional.*" The nonessential amino acids are those that can be reliably built by the body under all circumstances. There are 7 conditional amino acids that your body can make on its own under normal, healthy circumstances. However, when you are under a lot of physical stress due to illness or prolonged physical training, you may need to supplement them in your diet.

Neurotransmitters

Among the many molecules that the body makes from amino

acids are *neurotransmitters* which are chemical messengers in the brain. Remember learning about neurons, the main cells within the brain and nervous system, in Chapter 2? You may recall that neurons have dendrites, which receive messages, and axons, which send messages. Well, between the one neuron's axon and the next neuron's dendrite is a synapse, or space between neurons where chemical reactions take place to transmit messages; neurotransmitters are the tiny vehicles that carry these messages.

There are many diverse types of neurotransmitters, and they're all built within neurons from various building blocks, including amino acids from the protein sources you eat. Once built, they are stored at the end of the neuron's axon and wait to be released. When the right message is transmitted to the end of the axon (the axon terminal), the appropriate neurotransmitters are released into the synapse between neurons. When they are released, they trigger a chemical reaction that prompts the next neuron to send the message along the line to the next neuron, and so on. Along with the many different types of neurotransmitters, there is an equally large number of different chemical reactions that can take place, so we will not get into all of them here. However, it suffices to say that without neurotransmitters, your brain would not be able to send and receive messages.

Although you may have heard of many different neurotransmitters, you may not be aware of them. Some of the more well-known chemical messengers in the brain include dopamine, histamine serotonin, norepinephrine, and epinephrine (a.k.a. adrenaline). Others that you may be familiar with are insulin, oxytocin, prolactin, and beta-endorphin. The list goes on, but you get the idea. Each neurotransmitter has a specific message to convey, and without it, a specific function within the body cannot take place.

What Happens When You Do Not Eat Enough Protein?

Almost all the neurotransmitters are created from one or more amino acids, many of which come from the foods you eat. If you do not eat enough of the right foods, you may end up deficient in one or more neurotransmitters which can have a serious effect on your brain's function, especially if your diet is deficient for an extended period.

A good example of the effects of a deficiency can be seen in the neurotransmitter, serotonin. Serotonin is fairly well-known because of its role in the brain for controlling emotions. Generally, it helps to produce good sleeping patterns and acts as a mood booster, and research has shown that this chemical is generally linked to positive effects on mood and behavior, as well as living a longer life. Low levels of serotonin can cause depressive disorders, sleep disorders, anxiety, obesity, chronic pain, eating disorders, and alcohol abuse.

Psychiatrists will often prescribe medication to help with serotonin deficiency. Although these prescriptions cannot create more serotonin, they help keep the serotonin that is present from being reabsorbed by neurons, essentially making it available for longer. But, what if the solution to low serotonin could be found in the foods we eat instead of medication?

Serotonin is created, in part, from the amino acid, tryptophan, which is one of the essential amino acids that you must take in from your food. Although tryptophan has gotten a reputation as being the nutrient in turkey that makes you sleepy on Thanksgiving Day, turkey is not the only source of tryptophan, nor is it even the highest source of tryptophan that you can find. Some other rich sources of tryptophan are eggs yolks, cheese, soy products like tofu, and salmon. Can you imagine if, instead of sending you to the pharmacy, your psychiatrist sent you to the grocery store to boost your serotonin levels?

What About Protein and Dementia?

Since the essential amino acids play such a key role in healthy brain function, it makes sense that not eating enough protein may lead to an increased risk of developing dementia. Not too long ago, however, a specific study made headlines for claiming that a "low protein and high carbohydrate diet" might help ward off dementia, specifically Alzheimer's disease.

As compelling as these headlines might be, this study needs to be evaluated for its scientific accuracy as well as the implications of its results. First of all, the study was conducted on mice who were eating pellets of carefully engineered food with varying levels of protein and carbohydrates. Secondly, the protein in the pellets was derived from a dairy extract, not from lean meat or vegetable protein sources. Thirdly, the carbohydrate sources in the pellets were sugar and refined starches, which are generally bad for human bodies, especially the brain. Essentially, the mice were eating junk food. Although the results of the study showed that a higher intake of carbohydrates improved overall cognitive function in mice, the authors of the study even stated that their findings were inconsistent. Additionally, it is hard to imagine comparing any human diet to the junk ingredients that went into the pellets that the mice ate.

A study that was more scientifically sound took a look at *human* brain responses to different levels of protein in their diets, and it came up with different results. After looking at more than 500 adults who ate low, medium, and high levels of protein every day, they found that those who ate high levels of protein had a reduced risk of developing Alzheimer's disease. Specifically, the researchers studied levels of *amyloid beta* in the participants' brains. Amyloid beta is a precursor to the plaques that form in the brain in active Alzheimer's disease. They discovered that those who ate about 120 grams of protein daily had significantly lower levels of amyloid beta in their brains (12 times lower, to be exact) than those who ate around 50 grams of protein each day.

It is unclear what the role of protein is in the formation of amyloid beta, but a few different hypotheses surround the results of the study. For example, some scientists believe that the difference is due to the link between a high-protein diet and a reduced risk of heart disease or other cardiovascular diseases due to decreased blood pressure. Others believe that eating more protein prevents you from eating unhealthy fats and carbohydrates, some of which can be damaging to the brain. Whatever the reason, the results were clear.

Healthy Sources of Protein for Better Brain Function

Before you go out and buy the biggest cut of prime rib or ribeye steak that you can find, remember that the key is to find lean sources of protein. Red meat tends to be higher in saturated fat, which is not good for brain health; we'll go into the reasons for that in Part 3 of this guide.

Some excellent lean animal sources of complete protein are low-fat or fat-free dairy, eggs, fish, and poultry. The occasional lean, red meat is okay, as long as the portions are small and are only eaten a couple times a week. There are also a few excellent sources of vegan complete protein sources. These sources include pumpkin seeds, quinoa, buckwheat, soybeans, and chia seeds. You can also combine a whole grain with a legume to create a complete protein source. Examples of such combinations are beans and rice or barley and lentils.

If you are wondering how much protein you should get in a day, you may find many conflicting answers. The current official Recommended Dietary Allowance (RDA) is .36 grams of protein per pound of body weight, which comes out to about 56 grams for the average man or 46 grams for the average woman. Additionally, active people require more protein, and these amounts vary by activity levels, body sizes, and fitness goals. But, what about the study that said it's better to eat more than 100 grams per day?

Before you decide to consume 120 grams of protein every day, please discuss this decision with your doctor or a registered dietician. Certain health problems, like reduced kidney function, can make it dangerous to consume such high levels of protein.

Here is a guide to how much protein is in some healthy sources:

- 100 grams of chicken breast = 31 grams of protein
- 100 grams of salmon = 20 grams of protein
- 1 large egg = 6 grams of protein
- 8 ounces of Greek yogurt = 18 grams of protein (beware of added sugar in yogurt!)
- ¼ cup of pumpkin seeds = 3 grams of protein
- 1 cup of cooked barley = 23 grams of protein
- 1 cup of cooked lentils = 18 grams of protein
- 1 cup of cooked black beans = 39 grams of protein
- ½ cup of cooked quinoa = 12 grams of protein
- 100 grams of buckwheat flour = 13 grams of protein
- 1 cup of cooked soybeans (edamame) = 29 grams of protein
- 1 tablespoon of chia seeds = 3 grams of protein

This list could go on and on, but you get the idea. Find creative ways of incorporating healthy protein sources into your diet. For breakfast, you can eat 8 ounces of Greek yogurt with a tablespoon of chia seeds sprinkled in. At lunchtime, try adding beans or an egg to your salad, and don't forget to include fish or poultry (unless you are a strict vegetarian). If this is the case, a nice dish of red beans and rice might be just the ticket to a complete protein meal for you.

Next, we'll look at the essential role of healthy fats in your diet.

7

FABULOUS FAT

FAT HAS GAINED AN UNFORTUNATE REPUTATION IN RECENT DECADES. Everywhere you look in grocery stores; you can see products labeled with "reduced fat" or "fat-free" and many snacks are deemed "healthy" because of their low fat content. You may even feel guilty eating bacon or donuts because of the amount of fat in these foods.

While it is true that we need to limit certain types of food in our diets or avoid some of them altogether, we should not be so quick to dismiss *all* fat as evil and terrible for us. This is because certain types of fat are not only beneficial to the body, but they are utterly essential to maintaining the health of our brains.

The Role of Fat in the Body and Brain

Our bodies cannot produce certain types of fat on its own, and a certain amount of fat is completely necessary for it to be able to function. Some of the important functions of fat in the body include energy storage, insulation, assisting proteins as they do their jobs, acting as messengers, and starting important chemical reactions. Fat also helps to store certain essential vitamins, those that are called "*fat-soluble,*" which are vitamins D, K, E, and A. Although we get a certain amount of energy from sugar, much of our energy is stored in the form of fat, and we can access this energy whenever the immediate, available energy sources (from sugar) are depleted. Additionally, fat is a part of the structural make-up of many parts of our body including the brain.

Types of Fat

Before we go into more detail of what fat does in the brain, it's important to note the different types of fat that are available in our diets; these are *saturated fats, monounsaturated fats, polyunsaturated fats,* and *trans fats.* Additionally, fats have numerous carbon atoms chained together, with hydrogen atoms attached to them; all of these names describe the number of double bonds between the carbon atoms.

The more double bonds between carbon atoms, the less room there is for hydrogen. A chain of carbon atoms without double bonds (which, therefore, as much hydrogen as possible) is called *saturated fat.* Sources of saturated fat include animal fats found in dairy products like butter, milk, yogurt, and cheese. Other saturated fats are found in red meat and lard. Although these fats are important for energy storage, they should be limited in your diet which we'll get more into in Part 3 of this book.

Another type of fat that should be limited, or better yet, avoided altogether is *trans fat,* a.k.a. *trans fatty acids.* Trans fats are artificially produced by taking an unsaturated fat and adding hydrogen to it. Like unsaturated fats, these chains still have double bonds, but they bend in a way that makes it easy for a multitude of chains to stack together, which make it difficult for the body to break it down. Although there are a few natural animal sources of trans fats, most trans fatty acids that we eat today are artificially produced. The reason for this production is that trans fats are solid while at room temperature and tend to have a long shelf life. While this quality is beneficial for commercial food production for many reasons, ultimately, these fats should be avoided, which we will explain in further detail in Part 3. Trans fats are found in fried foods, margarine, and commercially baked foods, just to name a few sources.

Now that you've learned about the "bad" fats, it's time to talk about the brain-friendly sources of fat. One kind of "good" fat is *monounsaturated fat (MUFAs)*. These chains of carbon atoms contain one double bond, meaning there is one place in the chain that has fewer hydrogen atoms than possible. These fat sources are liquid at room temperature, but start to solidify at cooler temperatures. Olive oil and canola oils are both good examples of MUFAs.

The second type of "good" fat for the brain is *polyunsaturated fat (PUFAs)*. These chains of carbon atoms have more than one double bond, meaning there are multiple places where there are fewer hydrogen atoms than possible. Examples of these fats are *Omega-3 fatty acids*, which are found in fatty fish, nuts, and *Omega-6 fatty acids*. Other foods that are high in these include safflower oil, corn oil, and nuts like walnuts and pecans. In general, many foods have both Omega-3 and Omega-6 fatty acids, but the key is to find foods with higher concentrations of Omega-3's than Omega-6's. Omega-6's are important, but consuming too many of them has been linked to higher inflammation in the body. Together, Omega-3 and Omega-6 fatty acids are called *essential fatty acids* (EFAs).

The Role of PUFAs in the Brain

Although saturated fat is important to the rest of the body for energy storage, the brain cannot access any energy from fat. Thus, the fat that is important for the brain is structural. When the water content of the brain is not considered, this organ is made up of about 60 percent fat.

So, what is all of that fat doing in the brain? Well, when the brain is still forming, before a child is born and throughout childhood, essential fatty acids (EFAs) are critical for forming the actual structure of the brain, particularly during fetal and infant periods. This is especially true for Omega-3 fatty acids. Studies have shown that extra sources of specific Omega-3's is related to improved mental development in children. Since our bodies cannot create EFAs, we must rely on our diets to provide them.

After the brain structure is established and the brain has finished growing, EFAs continue to play important roles in adult brains. For example, they play a part in building the neurotransmitters mentioned in the previous chapter, and they are also essential for the immune system. These important fat sources also continue to help maintain the structure of the brain in adults, even after the brain is done actively growing. They help to keep the membranes (the outside edges) of neuron cells flexible so that the proteins within these cell membranes can continue to change shape when necessary. For example, whenever a neurotransmitter is released by one neuron, the proteins within the receiving neuron's dendrites must react to these neurotransmitters to communicate the message that the brain is trying to send. Ultimately, the changes in the cell membrane that fuel the brain's communication system are dependent on the existence of essential fatty acids in your diet.

If brain cells do not receive enough polyunsaturated fats or PUFAs, their membranes can become stiff and rigid, thus slowing down communication between cells or stopping communication altogether. As a result, a person's thoughts and reactions, voluntary or involuntary, become sluggish. This is why diets that are low in

PUFAs have been associated (via scientific studies) with brain problems such as chronic depression, hormone imbalances, chronic pain, poor memory abilities, and increased risks of neurodegenerative diseases like dementia.

Besides the cell membranes, the myelin sheaths that encase the axon terminals of neurons are also made up primarily of specialized essential fatty acids. As we mentioned in Chapter 2, the myelin sheath helps ensure the speed and strength of message transmission between neurons. Without it, cell communication breaks down. In a disease like multiple sclerosis (MS), the myelin sheath is attacked by the body's immune system. However, in a healthy body without an auto-immune issue, myelin sheaths depend on a steady diet of Omega-3 fatty acids to maintain their structure. Without this key dietary component, communication in the brain, and thus throughout the body's entire nervous structure, can be compromised.

Although EFAs are vital to the brain, there is one caveat, which is that it is possible to eat too much Omega-6 fatty acid. Omega-6 fats are important for brain function, but they can also cause inflammation in the body and brain. Because of the prevalence of foods cooked or fried with corn oil, safflower oil, soybean oil, along with several other sources of Omega-6 fatty acids, most Americans eat far more EFAs than are good for them. The key to a healthy balance of fats in your diet is to focus on consuming more sources of Omega-3 fatty acids. Health experts and neurologists recommend consuming a ratio of 4 Omega-6 for every 1 Omega 3 fatty acid. That's a 4:1 ratio, but most Americans consume a ratio of 12:1 or higher in favor of Omega-6's. This unbalanced ratio can help lead to cardiovascular problems and neurodegenerative diseases like Alzheimer's. Instead of the 4:1 ratio, some experts who study brain aging even suggest going as far as to suggest eating a ratio of 1:1 so that more Omega-3's can help protect the brain. Again, remember that you *must* consume some Omega-6's for optimal health, but they must be limited despite the fact that it is hard to avoid them.

The Role of Monounsaturated Fats in the Brain

Monounsaturated fatty acids (MUFAs) are another type of fat that the body needs. Like PUFAs, these are extremely important to maintaining optimal health and protecting your brain against damage and deterioration. One of the critical functions of MUFAs in your brain has to do with blood circulation. When you replace saturated fat with MUFAs, your total cholesterol levels drop, particularly your LDL levels, which are the "bad" type of cholesterol. Bad cholesterol clogs your arteries and can lead to circulatory problems and (oftentimes) causing heart attacks and strokes. Too much bad cholesterol can lead to decreased blood flow in your brain, resulting in a reduction in oxygen and nutrients that go to the neurons. Over time, if brain cells are starved of oxygen and nutrients long enough, significant damage can occur and contribute to serious problems like dementia.

On top of their contribution to healthy blood circulation, monounsaturated fats also have anti-inflammatory properties. Although inflammation is your body's method of fighting infection, chronic inflammation that occurs over a long period of time ends up damaging various parts of the body. Since inflammation contributes to most diseases, MUFAs are important in helping prevent many diseases. Regarding brain function, inflammation can be extremely detrimental. Research has shown that depression, along with other mood and psychotic disorders, is associated with inflammation on a cellular level within neurons. This microscopic inflammation can cause an imbalance of important neurotransmitters, such as serotonin, as discussed in the previous chapter.

Although various prescriptions can be used to fight the causes and symptoms of depression and other inflammation-based brain disorders, wouldn't it be nice to find the solution in your diet? As mentioned previously, too many Omega-6 fatty acids can promote unhealthy levels of inflammation. The same is true of too much saturated fat in your diet. Conversely, diets that are high in MUFAs have been repeatedly shown to reduce inflammation, thus helping to prevent heart and brain problems that are associated with long-term inflammation.

Another function of monounsaturated fats in your brain that is worth mentioning has to do with a neurotransmitter called acetylcholine, which is critical in functions such as memory and learning. Conversely, if your brain does not receive enough MUFA, less acetylcholine is produced. The lack of this important neurotransmitter leads to issues with memory that are associated with Alzheimer's disease and other forms of dementia.

Finally, monounsaturated fat sources are also rich in vitamin E, which is a powerful *antioxidant* that we need in our diet. Antioxidants like vitamin E are important to brain health because they help fight damage to the neurons that occurs as a part of the aging process. When oxygen molecules are broken down in the process of releasing energy from food, they lose electrons and become very unstable. These unstable molecules then search for stable molecules in healthy cells to pair with so that they can become stable again. Unfortunately, in this process of stabilization, they create more unstable molecules known as *free radicals*. As we get older, the number of free radicals produced within our cells increases, less energy is produced and our cells become more damaged. However, antioxidants like vitamin E help by donating electrons to deactivate these free radicals and keep them from damaging healthy cells.

Even though damage associated with aging is inevitable, the presence of certain toxins from pollution in our environment contributes to accelerated damage in the brain, which in turn can make us more at risk for dementia. Ultimately, in order to protect our brain cells from damage for as long as possible, we must include antioxidants like vitamin E in our diets.

Sources of PUFAs and MUFAs

Here are some foods that you should consider adding to your diet to make sure you get plenty of these EFAs:

Omega-3 Fatty Acids:

- Fatty fish, like wild-caught salmon, mackerel, tuna, sardines, and anchovies
- Chia seeds
- Flaxseed oil, flax seed meal and flax seeds
- Walnuts and Brazil nuts
- Avocados
- Hemp seeds and hemp seed oil
- Pumpkin seeds
- Sesame seeds

Omega-6 Fatty Acids:

- Flax seeds, including oil and meal from these seeds
- Grapeseed oil
- Pumpkin seeds and raw sunflower seeds
- Pine nuts
- Pistachios
- Hemp seeds and hemp seed oil

Note: corn, safflower and soybean oil are among oils that contain

Omega-6's, but because these are commercially refined, they often lack other nutrients and can contribute to too much inflammation.

- *Monounsaturated Fatty Acids:*
- Extra virgin olive oil, specifically true cold-pressed
- Avocados
- Olives
- Nuts, such as pistachios, pecans, macadamia nuts, almonds, and cashews

If you're wondering how much of each of these to incorporate into your diet, some good guides can be found in the MIND, DASH, and Mediterranean diets described in Chapter 3. Try substituting cold-pressed extra virgin olive oil as your main cooking oil and source of flavoring from fat. Eat fatty fish, particularly those low in mercury, 2 or 3 times per week. Snack on avocados, seeds, or nuts about five times a week, and try sprinkling chia seeds or flax seeds on your yogurt, oatmeal, soups, and salads. If you follow these suggestions and experiment with other healthy sources of fat mentioned above, you will be able to protect your brain from some of the damage that leads to dementia.

8

VIRTUOUS VITAMINS

OVER AND OVER, YOU'VE HEARD HOW IMPORTANT IT IS TO EAT YOUR fruits and vegetables. These powerful parts of the diet make countless contributions to good health, and protection of your brain's functions is no exception. The diets mentioned in Chapter 3 include a variety of vegetables and fruits for a good reason, as plant parts contain vitamins and minerals that are indispensable when it comes to preventing dementia. In this section, you'll learn about the different vitamins, minerals, and other chemicals that are important for your brain's health and which fruits, vegetables, and other foods can provide them.

Plants contain a powerful group of nutrients called *phytonutrients*. These nutrients are chemicals produced within various plants to protect the plant itself from different threats, including insect predation, bacteria, UV rays, and fungal infections among other things. Although nature did not produce phytonutrients to benefit those who eat them, we can take advantage of these natural super-nutrients by consuming the plants that contain them. Not only do they benefit the plants that create them, but they can provide many different health benefits for our body parts, particularly the brain.

Among some of the most critical phytonutrients are vitamins. This chapter breaks down the vitamins and explains the roles they each play in brain health, as well as the food sources where each vitamin can be found. As you'll see, there are one or two vitamins that do *not* come from plants, but the overwhelming majority of vitamins can be found in plant and animal sources. Animal sources that contain many of these vitamins are considered *secondary sources,* meaning they contain phytonutrients because they once consumed plants that were sources of the vitamins.

Neuroprotective Vitamins

Many different vitamins are useful for the production of energy in the brain as well as other processes that contribute to your powerful mental abilities. Vitamins can be divided into *water-soluble* and *fat-soluble* vitamins, both of which are important regarding brain function. Water-soluble vitamins include the B vitamin groups, and vitamin C. These are hard to overdose on because any excesses are flushed out of the body via urine. Conversely, it is possible to take in too much of some fat-soluble vitamins such as vitamins D, E, K, and A because they are stored in the body's fat. Too much of these can be harmful to the body, so it's important to watch out for signs concerning vitamin overdose.

The B Group Vitamins

Later on, we'll discuss the importance of glucose to the brain for energy. Without getting into the benefits of glucose itself, it's important for you to know that B vitamins help with to convert glucose to energy. They also help make neurotransmitters assist with the transport of oxygen in the brain and help protect the brain from toxins and oxidants. A regular intake of these vitamins in your diet is required for maximum brain function and for protection against damage that can lead to dementia or other brain problems.

Vitamin B1 (Thiamin)

Thiamin can only be stored in small quantities in the body, so you must take it in regularly, otherwise, you could suffer from poor memory, confusion, and irritability, and that's just the beginning. If you are severely deficient in thiamin, your brain can be permanently damaged. Research has shown improvement in various brain-linked behavior problems such as anxiety disorders, hyperactivity, and learning disabilities when people are treated with thiamine supplements.

You can find vitamin B1 (thiamin) in plant sources such as bell peppers, lettuce, zucchini, potatoes, asparagus, mushrooms, watercress, and cabbage. You can also find it in nuts and legumes, such as peas, which have been discussed in the protein and fat sections of this guide. Brown rice, pork, and eggs are additional sources of B1.

Vitamin B2 (Riboflavin)

Riboflavin plays many key roles in the body, and since it is an essential nutrient, it must be included in the diet because the body cannot make it. It is especially important for energy production. For the brain, in particular, it is required in order to create ATP, which provides energy for muscle contractions and the impulse messages sent by nerves, and for the overall health of the nerves within your brain and throughout the entire nervous system.

Consuming enough riboflavin in your diet supports healthy brain function, including memory and critical thinking abilities. Without enough B2, you may suffer from depression, migraines, and an increased risk of dementia. Signs that you are extremely deficient in B2 include fatigue, a sore or swollen tongue, sore throat, dry and/or cracked lips, sensitive and bloodshot eyes, and overall numbness.

Dietary sources of riboflavin include mushrooms, cabbage, watercress, asparagus, broccoli, tomatoes, and bean sprouts. Dairy products, pumpkin and pumpkin seeds, and almonds also contain riboflavin.

Vitamin B3 (Niacin)

Niacin is one of the key players in the production of energy of the mitochondria of your cells. As mentioned previously, the mitochondria are considered the "powerhouses" of the cell because they are responsible for breaking down nutrients and making energy for the cells to use in other processes. Your neurons have mitochondria, so niacin is just as essential to them as it is to the other cells in your body. It is perhaps even more critical because when energy in the brain runs low, your thoughts, memory, and reaction times become sluggish.

Additionally, niacin plays a part in nerve cell growth and repair when they are damaged. This vitamin also helps to balance blood sugar, which contributes to your overall energy levels too. Niacin also helps to lower LDL (bad) cholesterol and raise HDL (good) cholesterol, which improves circulation throughout the body as well as the brain.

People who are extremely deficient in B3 experience fatigue, sleep disorders, anxiety, depression, confusion, and have trouble with memory recall. Research has found reduced levels of niacin in patients who have dementia, so this deficiency may ultimately lead to the development of neurological disorders including Alzheimer's if left untreated. Similarly, other studies have linked vitamin B3 supplementation through diet to a decreased risk of age-related dementia.

You can find niacin in a variety of vegetables and fruits including cauliflower, zucchini, various squashes, mushrooms, cabbage, tomatoes, asparagus, a variety of green leafy vegetables, prunes, figs, and potatoes. Other sources of B3 are meat, fish, whole grain cereals, pine nuts, tahini, sunflower seeds, peas, and peanuts.

Vitamin B5 (Pantothenic acid)

Pantothenic acid is essential to your mental alertness and memory functions. Like the other B vitamins we've discussed, it is important for the production of energy and the overall function of your brain and nerves. In Chapter 7, you learned that monounsaturated fats play a part in the production of the neurotransmitter acetylcholine. Vitamin B5 is also needed for this neurotransmitter to be made. Without enough acetylcholine, people can experience brain "fog", a general term for lack of focus along with problems with memory and learning abilities. This vitamin also contributes to the production of other neurotransmitters, such as serotonin and epinephrine, which are important for regulating your mood and alertness, as well as reacting quickly and appropriately to stress. It is similar to vitamin B3 in that it also helps lower LDL cholesterol and ward off damage to the nerves.

Signs that you are not getting enough pantothenic acid can include anxiety and depression which can represent a lowered ability to cope with stress. Other symptoms include fatigue, muscle cramps, and a poor ability to concentrate. Ultimately, chronic stress and anxiety from a deficiency of vitamin B5 can lead to long-term damage to your brain which may show up in the form of Parkinson's disease or Alzheimer's disease. In less severe cases, mild to moderate memory loss or brain fog can occur.

Fruits and vegetables that contain B5 include tomatoes, broccoli, celery, squash, watercress, alfalfa sprouts, avocados, strawberries, and mushrooms. You can also find B5 in legumes such as lentils and peas, meat, and whole wheat bread.

Vitamin B6 (Pyridoxine)

Like vitamin B5, pyridoxine is necessary for building the neurotransmitters serotonin and norepinephrine. As such, it is a natural antidepressant and helps the body maintain a healthy immune system. This vitamin also contributes to the production of melatonin, which helps you maintain a healthy sleep cycle. It is vital to the development of a healthy brain in children and the continued healthy function of the brain in adults.

Without enough B6 in your diet, you may experience poor memory abilities, depression, irritability, fatigue, and anxiety. Additionally, some studies have provided evidence that getting enough of this vitamin can help to reduce your risk of cognitive decline including memory loss, stroke, and Alzheimer's disease.

Foods that you should eat to get enough B6 are bell peppers, onions, asparagus, cabbage, broccoli, cauliflower, bananas, and watercress. Additional sources include red kidney beans, lentils, nuts, lean meats, and fish.

Vitamin B7 (Biotin)

Within the body, biotin helps to break down carbohydrates and fat into usable energy. It is also responsible for helping the body control blood sugar levels and maintains overall healthy nerve functions. It also helps the function of many enzymes (necessary participants of chemical reactions) in the brain and throughout the body. Additionally, it is thought to play an important role in the production of the myelin sheath around axons. It is possible that biotin may have a part in the treatment of MS in the future.

Deficiency of B7 is rare, but it can occur. Symptoms of a biotin deficiency may include issues with the nervous system, dry skin, fatigue, and brittle hair.

Biotin is found in sweet potatoes, leafy green vegetables, and nuts and seeds. Other sources of B7 include eggs, pork, salmon, and dairy products.

Vitamin B9 (Folate)

Folate is also essential to brain health for several reasons. For example, it is required for the delivery of oxygen to the brain, which is important for clear thinking abilities. Additionally, it supports the concentrations of Omega-3 fatty acids in the brain, which are important to the function of your nerves and brain. Along with other B vitamins, folate assists with the production of important neurotransmitters. Folate is critical in prenatal care because it contributes to the growth of fetal nervous systems. Getting enough folate, or its synthetic form (folic acid) is important for preventing congenital disabilities that affect the nervous system.

Low amounts of vitamin B9 have been shown to cause an increased risk of stroke, memory loss, depression, congenital disabilities, and miscarriages. Severely low amounts of B9 in adults has also been linked to psychiatric disorders and mood instability.

Vitamin B9 can be found in parsley, spinach, broccoli, asparagus, beets, bananas, citrus fruits, and sprouts. Other non-vegetable sources of this vitamin include hazelnuts, cashews, walnuts, sesame seeds, and legumes.

Vitamin B12 (Cyanocobalamin)

Vitamin B12 is critically important to brain function. Like vitamin

B7, it helps with the formation and maintenance of the myelin sheath, which is important for message transmission between your brain's neurons. It also helps protect the neurons from damage.

Because of its importance to the myelin sheath, deficiency in B12 can have severe neurological effects, especially in older people. Still, people younger than age 40 can be affected by B12 deficiencies, though they are rarely. Diseases of the spinal cord and nerves, as well as muscle weaknesses, can result from a lack of B12 in the diet. Additional cognitive effects include confusion, memory loss, disorientation, and dementia. Other psychiatric problems have also been known to result from a deficiency in B12.

Unlike other B vitamins, vitamin B12 is mainly found in animal foods. Thus, it is important that vegans and vegetarians incorporate a B12 supplement into their diets because it is so very essential to the brain!

Vitamin C (Ascorbic acid)

Vitamin C is a very small, water-soluble nutrient that can pass through the blood-brain barrier very easily. It is found in extremely high concentrations in brain tissue compared to other areas in the body, and it has a couple of very important functions there. One of them is to contribute to the creation of neurotransmitters, much like some of the B vitamins, and it has a direct impact on the strength and speed of electric impulses in your brain. Another essential function of vitamin C in the brain is that it acts as an antioxidant. Remember learning about vitamin E as an antioxidant in Chapter 7? In a similar way, vitamin C also plays this role as a stabilizer of damaging free radicals in our brain. As a result, getting plenty of vitamin C from your diet is very important if you want to protect your brain from oxidative damage.

If you do not get enough vitamin C in your diet, you may experience poor wound healing, fatigue, depression, low immunity, and easy bruising. Vitamin C deficiency is also directly related to increased damage to aging brains which can result in increased rates of cognitive impairment.

You can find vitamin C in many plant sources, including bell peppers, citrus fruits, melons, potatoes, broccoli, strawberries, cabbage, tomatoes, watercress, and kiwi fruit.

Vitamin A

Vitamin A is a fat-soluble vitamin, meaning that it is stored in your body's fat and getting too much this nutrient can be harmful. Plant sources that contain this vitamin also contain beta-carotene, which is a precursor to the vitamin. Much like vitamin C, it acts as an antioxidant that helps fight damage from free radicals, and it is important to the functioning of your immune system. When the brain is still growing in fetuses and children, getting plenty of vitamin A is essential to the formation of healthy brain cells.

Recent research has suggested that vitamin A also plays a key role in memory formation and retrieval, although further research needs to be done. Older people who do not have enough vitamin A have been proven to typically experience memory and other cognitive problems. Additionally, even a slight deficiency in vitamin A intake can increase one's risk of developing Alzheimer's by a significant amount. Sometimes, giving people with memory problems a vitamin A supplement has helped them recover a certain amount of their recall abilities.

Other research has shown that *too much* vitamin A can also cause problems, especially in terms of the immune system and production of energy in cells. Too much vitamin A might also act as a type of fuel for the growth of blood vessels in tumors. This research shows that a careful balance of vitamin A is likely needed for you to maintain optimal health.

Because it is possible to get too much vitamin A and other fat-soluble vitamins, experts warn against taking vitamin A supplements, which usually contain huge doses of these. Instead, you should get your vitamin A from food which can be found in animal sources like meat, fish, poultry, eggs, and dairy products. Fruits and vegetables that contain beta-carotene include sweet potatoes, carrots, apricots, bell peppers, papayas, pumpkin, green leafy vegetables, tangerines, asparagus, and tomatoes.

Vitamin D (calciferol)

Although we have labeled D a "vitamin," it is technically a hormone because our bodies produce it from 2 different components when we are exposed to sunlight. These two components are D2 and D3. Within the brain, vitamin D stimulates substances called neurotrophins, which help to regulate the functions of neurons within adult brains. Neurotrophins also stimulate the growth and differentiation of immature neurons within the growing brains of children.

Additionally, vitamin D is important in the creation of neurotransmitters for sending messages between cells in the nervous system. It is also involved in the growth of nerves. Recent studies have shown that this hormone helps protect neurons from damage.

Research into vitamin D deficiencies has shown that it is critical to optimal brain health. Without enough vitamin D in your system, you may run the risk of slower reasoning and critical thinking. These slow cognitive functions may ultimately lead to the development of dementia as we age. Some studies on animals have shown that vitamin D may help reduce the amount of the protein *amyloid* in the brain. Amyloid can lead to the plaques that form in active Alzheimer's disease. More research is needed, but evidence may show how vitamin D can prevent Alzheimer's in people who are at high-risk for the disease. Additionally, too little vitamin D in a fetus, infant, or child diet may lead to impaired brain development and lifelong deficiencies in brain function.

Vitamin D can be found in cold-pressed vegetable oils as well as animal products such as eggs, butter, and fish which are especially rich in this nutrient. However, it is almost impossible to get enough vitamin D from your diet alone if you do not receive sufficient sunshine each day. For this reason, medical experts recommend that people who live in the Northern Hemisphere take a vitamin D3 supplement. 5,000 to 8,000 IU daily is recommended for adults who do not have enough D in their blood. For growing infants in northern climates, a supplement of 800 IU daily is recommended. Before taking vitamin D supplements, talk to your doctor. He or she will likely recommend checking a blood sample to see if you have adequate levels of this hormone.

Vitamin E (Tocopherol)

You've already learned a bit about vitamin E via the discussion of monounsaturated fats, so you know that it is a powerful antioxidant, like vitamins A and C. By neutralizing free radicals in brain cells, vitamin E helps to protect against damage and ensure that messages can transmit quickly and accurately throughout the nervous system. Additionally, the liver uses vitamin E to build molecules that deliver Omega-3 fatty acids to the brain. As you may recall, Omega-3's are critical to brain health, so a lack of vitamin E leads to a secondary reduction of these essential fatty acids in the brain. As a result, neuron cell membranes become inflexible and less able to transmit messages to each other. As a result of this deficiency, communication in the brain and nervous system may begin to fail.

Just as with deficiencies in vitamins A and C, having too little vitamin E has been linked to various levels of dementia, from mild cognitive impairment to full-blown Alzheimer's disease. Other side effects of a vitamin E deficiency can be easy exhaustion, bruising, decreased muscle tone, and slow wound healing.

Although vitamin E is a fat-soluble vitamin, thus far, research has not been able to definitively prove that it is possible to take too much of this nutrient. So, unlike vitamin A, you can most likely safely take a supplement of vitamin E. However, your best bet is to find natural sources first. Besides the cold-pressed vegetable oils like extra virgin olive oil, vitamin E is also found in a few other plant products. These sources include sweet potatoes and green leafy vegetables, along with nuts and seeds, legumes like beans and peas, oats, and whole grain cereals and bread. Additionally, a great non-plant source of vitamin E is fish.

Vitamin K

Vitamin K is our fourth and final fat-soluble vitamin, and its well-known primary role has been in blood clotting and the formation of bones. However, newer research has also linked it to brain function. Just as in bones, vitamin K helps to monitor and ensure a healthy level of calcium in the brain, which may have something to do with whether or not Alzheimer's can develop. Newly emerging evidence shows that a low level of vitamin K in the brain may contribute to a high risk of Alzheimer's disease; however, more research is needed in this area.

There are two natural forms of healthy vitamin K, known as KI and K2. A third synthetic form (K3) can be harmful and is best avoided. You can consume KI via many different plants including brussel sprouts, kale, peas, asparagus, broccoli, cauliflower, cabbage, lettuce, swiss chard, collard greens, and watercress. It can also be found in vegetable oil. K2 comes from the good bacteria that live in your gut. You may need to take a probiotic or increase your intake of fermented foods such as kimchi, sauerkraut, yogurt with active cultures, kefir, and tempeh if you do not have a healthy digestive function. If you do have a healthy digestive tract, K2 can also be found in animal products like cheeses, meats, and butter.

Why Not Just Take a Supplement?

You may be wondering why, if these vitamins are so essential to brain health and the prevention or development of dementia, you cannot just take a supplement. It would be so much easier than seeking out all of these different food sources, right?

For one thing, you have learned that there are some cases in which it is possible to take too much of a vitamin, as is the case of vitamin A. In the case of some underlying health conditions, other vitamins, when taken in the mega-doses found in supplements, can also be harmful. For example, in cases of liver damage or kidney disease, too much vitamin K can be toxic.

Secondly, vitamins are much more easily absorbed from food than from supplements. This is because dietary supplements are not regulated like medications, but rather like food. As a result, they can be sold to the public without having been tested for their purity or effectiveness! It's a little scary to think that your multivitamin might not contain what it says it contains or that there may be additives that are not listed on the label.

Many times, vitamins require other vitamins to be as effective as possible. There is a good reason that nature packages multiple vitamins into one food – because these nutrients do the most good when they are together. So, when you just take one type of vitamin (like vitamin C or B6) alone, you may not be getting the desired benefits.

Finally, plant and animal sources of vitamins contain more nutrients than just vitamins; they also contain protein and fat as we've already discussed. Additionally, you can find beneficial fiber in plants. Every day, scientists are discovering more nutrients from plants that have yet to be packaged into a convenient pill form. So, when you try to fill in nutritional gaps from your diet with supplements, you are missing out on unknown health benefits from plants, not to mention the fun of trying new flavors! We simply cannot replicate the goodness of nature into a tiny pill or convenient powder.

9

MARVELOUS MINERALS

ALONG WITH VITAMINS, MINERALS ARE OTHER ESSENTIAL NUTRIENTS needed for the brain to function at peak health and to help keep you feeling sharp. The body does not require them in the quantities that vitamins are needed, but they are still just as important. Minerals are categorized into *major minerals*, which are needed in larger quantities, and *trace elements*, which are needed the body in lesser amounts.

Here, we will look at the major minerals and trace elements that are critical to incorporate into your diet and the role that each of them plays in protecting your brain.

Major Minerals

Calcium

You may recall that we ended our discussion of vitamins with vitamin K, which regulates the levels of calcium within the bones and the brain. You most likely remember learning about the importance of calcium for healthy bones, since, as children, many of us were instructed to drink our milk because it contained calcium for building strong bones. However, we were probably never taught about what calcium does in the brain.

In and around the neurons of the brain, calcium atoms exist in the form of *ions*, which are forms of atoms that have an electrical charge because they have lost or gained electrons. These calcium ions have the important task of joining with proteins in the cell membrane to tell the cell that a certain message has been delivered to that cell.

On the outside of a neuron, there are more calcium ions than on the inside of a neuron, and the difference between these two amounts of ions causes a difference in electrical charge across the neuron's membrane. This difference is called a *gradient*. If a tiny change takes place in the gradient, meaning that too many calcium ions have entered a cell, a healthy brain cell can detect this change and correct it by pumping some of the ions back outside where they wait for another message to arrive.

The mechanism that pumps calcium ions out of the cell depends on specific proteins. If these proteins do not exist or are sluggish, too much calcium can build up inside a neuron, ultimately killing that neuron. In aging neurons of the brain, these proteins that drive the calcium pump sometimes no longer exist or act very slow.

The slowness or non-existence of the proteins that pump calcium ions across cell membranes has been linked to Alzheimer's disease. Scientists have hypothesized that one of the processes that lead to Alzheimer's disease has to do with the DNA that codes for these calcium pump proteins. Older neurons seem to stop making these proteins, which leads to stressed and dying neurons that have too much calcium.

This theory about too much calcium in brain cells leading to

Alzheimer's may lead you to believe that calcium is bad for the brain cells; however, it is the exact opposite. Calcium is critical for transmitting messages in the brain cells, but the breakdown of the protein is to blame for the problems.

Scientists have yet to arrive at a definitive way to restore the proteins that pump calcium ions in neurons, but there are a few ideas that have proven helpful thus far. One of these is lowering your calorie intake unless you are already at a healthy weight. Studies have shown that eating less overall helps the brain keep the right amount of calcium ions inside its neurons for longer, thus keeping more neurons alive for longer.

Another helpful aid might be found in the supplement ginseng. More research is needed to be done, but ginseng may be helpful in aiding the calcium pump proteins and keeping cells from getting over-stressed by too much calcium. Based on this, it would not hurt to take a ginseng supplement! Finally, antioxidants are also very helpful in increasing the energy level of cells, including the activity of the pump proteins. You have already learned of the antioxidant vitamins C and E. Additional antioxidants can be found in berries and green teas, so feel free to enjoy these helpful additions to your diet.

Make sure you keep an adequate level of calcium in your diet to keep your brain and nerves functioning well. Calcium is present in many foods, and adding a supplement is often unnecessary. You can get enough calcium in your diet by eating plenty of green leafy vegetables, almonds, broccoli, cabbage, prunes, sesame seeds, pumpkin seeds, legumes, and figs. Additionally, dairy milk or vitamin-D fortified dairy alternatives, like soy milk or almond milk provide a nice boost of this nutrient.

As with other vitamins and minerals, you can get too much calcium with some supplements. To make sure you get no more than 1,000 to 1,200 mg per day, take a supplement with 500 to 700 mg of calcium, and aim to get the rest of your calcium from food. An excessive amount of calcium (3,000 mg per day or more) can lead to problems like depression, headaches, and exhaustion.

Potassium

Another major essential mineral is potassium which has a few different roles in the brain's function. One of its jobs is to help transmit messages from the brain to the smooth muscles of the digestive organs, telling them to contract so that food can be digested properly. It has a similar function in relaying messages between the brain and lungs, instructing them to perform the muscle contractions crucial to breathing. In the case of the message transmission to the digestive system and lungs, potassium acts much like the calcium ions described in the previous section. In other words, the movement of potassium ions back and forth across the membranes of nerve cells stimulates the transmission of signals between neurons. As a result, nerve cells would not be able to communicate important messages very well without potassium, leading to problems with digestion and breathing.

Besides the importance to your ability to digest food and breathe deeply, potassium has also been linked to your memory abilities. It has been proven to improve the ability to learn and recall information, even in healthy people who do not have dementia. Additionally, potassium helps reduce the amounts of free radicals in your brain, like the antioxidants we have previously discussed.

Studies have proven that people who have low blood potassium levels can suffer from overall brain "fog" in addition to the loss of memory recall and overall confusion. This reduction of memory abilities is often reversible through simple supplementation of potassium. To keep your memory sharp as you get older it is important for you to get enough potassium each day!

If your blood has been tested for potassium level and the result was low, you may benefit from a supplement, but it's best to check with your doctor first. The overall adult recommendation for potassium intake is 4.7 g each day. You can find potassium in several foods, including avocados, sweet potatoes, spinach, dairy and citrus fruits.

Beware of too much potassium, though, because if you supplement your diet with dangerous levels of potassium, you may end up with kidney disease or arrhythmia of the heart. Both conditions can be deadly, so you must consult with your doctor before taking a potassium supplement.

Magnesium

Recent research has revealed that magnesium is an essential nutrient for keeping a youthful brain. It assists the antioxidant vitamin E and also helps to reduce free radicals by itself. Moreover, it has been shown to maintain healthy neurons. The result of adequate magnesium directly impacts your ability to learn and remember important information.

Additionally, magnesium plays a part in emotional regulation by keeping the excessive excitatory activity of the nervous system in check. Magnesium helps neurons release the neurotransmitter gamma-aminobutyric acid (GABA), which is essential for relaxing the mind. All of these different functions show that this mineral is extremely critical in regulating your entire nervous system.

Additionally, lab research has shown that not getting enough magnesium reduces the brain's ability to form new connections between neurons. Neurons form new connections when we learn, so when we lose this ability, we are unable to learn or retain new information. The ability to form new connections in the brain is called its *plasticity*, and lowered plasticity is a key sign of neurodegenerative diseases like Alzheimer's.

Besides memory and learning issues, additional problems associated with insufficient magnesium are poor concentration, irritability, unstable and overreactive emotions, being easily startled, fatigue, and difficulty sleeping. All of these symptoms are closely linked to the roles that magnesium plays in overall brain and nerve function.

Fortunately, studies have also shown that the supplementation of magnesium can actually reverse some of these symptoms, including reduced memory abilities. At first, researchers discovered that traditional magnesium supplements are not absorbed well by the brain, but they had a breakthrough when they were able to develop a new form of magnesium supplement, called *magnesium-L-threonate*. Unlike many synthesized versions of vitamins and minerals, which are often ineffective or even harmful, this one has been shown to be helpful as it is readily absorbed into the brain.

In lab studies on animals, cognitive abilities were improved by supplementation of this form of magnesium. Evidence has also shown that human cognitive abilities may also benefit from this supplement, but more research is needed to support this evidence. Based on experiments done on mice, it is possible that supplementing Alzheimer's disease patients with magnesium-L-threonate may help to slow or reverse the disease, at least temporarily.

Magnesium-L-threonate supplements *are* available for purchase in stores and online, but I cannot stress enough that you must communicate with your doctor before taking it as they may be able to recommend a specific brand or potency or even advise you about whether or not you are a good candidate for magnesium supplementation. Fortunately, this is a nutrient that does not typically cause serious symptoms in the case of overdose, though you may experience diarrhea and vomiting.

Natural sources of magnesium are plentiful and harmless and include nuts like almonds, cashews, pecans, and Brazil nuts. Other good plant sources are pumpkin seeds, spinach, Swiss chard, cooked beans, raisins, garlic, quinoa, and green peas. Fatty fish like halibut, wild-caught salmon, and mackerel are high in magnesium, too.

Sodium

Since salt is often demonized as the enemy, especially when it comes to your cardiovascular health, some people are amazed to discover that it is also an essential nutrient. For example, in your brain, it plays a role similar to calcium and potassium – that is, it is important for the transmission of specific messages.

However, unlike calcium and potassium, it is almost impossible to get too little of this essential mineral, especially with the modern American diet. Most health experts warn us about the dangers of taking in too much sodium because too much sodium in the brain has been linked to memory problems and difficulty with other critical thinking skills. These symptoms can even become severe enough to be considered dementia.

Technically, it is possible to have too little sodium in your body compared to the water level, but health conditions typically cause this. Very rarely, drinking too much water can cause this imbalance, but most people will never have this problem!

It is critical to limit your sodium intake by checking the labels of any prepackaged foods that you eat. Per the American Heart Association, you should try to eat no more than 1,500 mg of sodium each day, with an absolute upper limit of 2,300 mg each day. Most sodium in our diets comes from pre-packaged foods, whether they are canned, boxed or frozen. Restaurant foods can also be a problem when it comes to too much sodium. So, the fresher the foods you purchase and prepare yourself, the healthier your sodium intake will be. Some natural sources of the salty flavors you crave include olives, beets, celery, and cabbage. The function of your brain depends on you paying attention to how much sodium is in the foods you are eating.

Chloride

The last major essential mineral we'll discuss is chloride. Like sodium, potassium, and calcium, this mineral is important for the transmission of impulses across cell membranes in the brain and throughout the nervous system.

Ingesting too much chloride is extremely dangerous for the body, but it is also very rare. To have dangerously high levels of chloride in your body, you would need to take in inordinately high amounts of salt in your diet, since table salt is sodium chloride. Other causes of high chloride are generally related to health problems or the use of certain prescription drugs over long periods of time.

Like with sodium, it is difficult to get too little chloride in your diet due to the prevalence of salt in our foods. However, some good natural sources of chloride are rye (whole, not processed), olives, sea salt, and seaweed.

Trace Elements

We need these minerals in very small amounts, and too much of some of these can be dangerous for the brain and the rest of the nervous system.

.   .   .

Chromium

This element is important to maintaining stable blood sugar levels, making it extremely important to brain function, since glucose fuels the brain. If chromium is in short supply, you may experience dizziness or irritability in between meals, drowsiness, or extreme thirst. Chromium also plays a role in building fatty acids and cholesterol, both of which are important to brain structure and function.

In a study of older adults with declining memories, supplementation of chromium was found to improve their overall cognitive abilities, including memory. These results show that chromium may be helpful in protecting against or even reversing early signs of dementia.

Besides supplements, chromium can be found in rye bread, apples, cornmeal, whole grain bread and cereal, tomatoes, potatoes, and romaine lettuce. It is hard to overdose on chromium, but excessive supplementation can lead to stomach pain, low blood sugar, or even damage to the kidneys or liver. As in all cases, consult your doctor before taking a supplement.

Copper

Copper is another nutrient that plays a critical role in the development of children's brains, although copper continues to be useful for adults because it is needed for the formation of various proteins that are important for brain function.

However, copper can be damaging in excessive amounts as too much copper can cause oxidative stress on brain cells due to the formation of free radicals. The brain has mechanisms in place for maintaining appropriate levels of copper, but the failure of these mechanisms puts the brain in danger of neurodegenerative problems, such as Alzheimer's disease.

It is difficult to get too little copper because it is widely available in many foods. Good, natural sources of copper include sesame seeds, sunflower seeds, macadamia nuts, cashews, lentils, garbanzo beans, and avocados. Excessive copper can be caused by contaminated water, so it is important to know whether your tap water has excessive copper. Additionally, cooking with copper pans or drinking water that flows through copper pipes is not recommended and is dangerous to the health of your brain.

Iodine

Iodine is another trace element that is essential to the formation of the brain in infants and children. Iodine deficiency during pregnancy or early development after birth has been shown to cause mental retardation, stunted physical growth, and difficulties in speech and hearing. Iodine is also essential to the function of the thyroid, which is important to the metabolism. Therefore, in adults whose brains are fully formed, insufficient iodine can cause a sluggish metabolism, dry skin and hair, depression, and difficulty concentrating.

In developed countries like the United States, iodine deficiency is not generally an issue because it is now added to table salt. Salt that has added iodine is labeled "iodized," in case you are unsure if your salt has it. However, if you have a diet that is completely devoid of table salt, some good alternative sources of iodine include seaweed, dairy products, whole grain products, fish, and shrimp. Fruits and vegetables also often contain iodine if they were grown in soil or fertilizer that contained this element.

Supplementation of iodine is not generally recommended, except under medical care for certain health problems. Too much iodine can negatively impact thyroid function, and an extremely high dose can even cause coma. If you are uncertain if you are getting enough iodine, discuss your concerns with your doctor.

Iron

The trace element iron is yet another essential nutrient for brain function. It's roles in the brain have to do with building important neurotransmitters and myelin, the protective covering of axons. As a result, insufficient iron can lead to brain cells being unable to send and receive messages. Iron deficiencies have an especially detrimental effect on the developing brains of infants, children, and adolescents, who can suffer from reduced cognitive function as a result of iron-poor diets. Sometimes this damage to the brain is irreversible. Iron deficiency in adults can also cause cognitive impairment, including fatigue, insomnia, confusion, and depression. Interestingly, iron deficiency has also been linked to psychological problems like ADHD and developmental disorders.

The first line of defense against iron deficiency is via the foods we eat. It is important to get a good mix of plant and animal sources of iron because these have two different forms of iron. Vegetation that contains iron includes pumpkin seeds, almonds, cashews, Brazil nuts, tofu, walnuts, dates, pecans, whole grain foods, and green leafy vegetables. Excellent animal sources of iron are meat and fish.

If too much iron is consumed via supplementation, this can cause problems for brain function as well. Research within the last decade has linked the accumulation of iron in the brain to neurodegenerative diseases like Parkinson's and Alzheimer's diseases. As a result, you should try and get your iron from food, and only use supplements if your doctor prescribes them. Excessive iron can also be found in well water, but it is typically not a problem in city water. So, if you drink well water, be sure to test for excessive iron and use an appropriate filter.

. . .

Manganese

The trace element manganese is also important in the early development of brains and nerves as it is needed for the production of energy in all cells, including neurons. It also plays the part of antioxidant molecules, so it helps to protect brain cells from damage due to free radicals.

Healthy brain and nerve function depend on adequate manganese in the diet, and low manganese has been related to seizure disorders and possibly to autism. Studies on the role of manganese in brain function showed that higher blood levels of manganese in children were related to higher IQ and better overall cognitive function. However, there is a limit to this relationship as excessive manganese can cause behavior problems in children due to its effect on the brain.

Additionally, getting enough manganese in the diet may help prevent Alzheimer's disease, but more research is needed to prove this relationship. For now, it is known that blood tests of Alzheimer's patients show significantly lower manganese levels than healthy people of similar ages.

Most people are in no danger of manganese deficiency because sufficient amounts can be found in many fruits and vegetables such as berries, pineapple, grapes, beets, and celery. Other plant sources of manganese include oats, nuts, and seeds.

Certain people are at risk of too much manganese in their blood, particularly infants, children, and patients with low iron levels, liver disease, kidney failure, or preexisting neurological disorders. Too much manganese in the brain can keep mitochondria, the energy producers, from functioning correctly. Like low manganese levels, excessive manganese has also been linked to Alzheimer's disease. Therefore, getting just enough manganese without overloading on it seems to be important for optimal protection of the brain.

If you are concerned that you are vulnerable to too much or too little manganese, talk to your healthcare provider.

Molybdenum

Molybdenum is yet another element that is essential to brain function in tiny amounts. Deficiency is very rare because very little is needed, and it is easy to get from food. However, a deficiency in this element can lead to too little uric acid in the blood which has the potential to cause neurological diseases like multiple sclerosis, Alzheimer's disease, Huntington's disease, and Parkinson's disease.

Molybdenum is available in many foods, but some of the best sources are whole grain bread and cereals, pumpkin seeds, peanuts, beans, lentils, and tomatoes.

Selenium

Selenium, another trace element, is needed for producing the antioxidant glutathione. Glutathione is produced in the nerve cells, and it plays an important part in fighting damage from oxidative stress. Ultimately, selenium is also involved with memory and critical thinking skills.

In patients who have Alzheimer's and Parkinson's diseases, decreasing selenium levels were associated with declining mental abilities. Future studies may help scientists to understand the cause and effect relationship in this association.

Brazil nuts contain over 500 micrograms of selenium per ounce, and since the recommended daily allowance of selenium is 200 micrograms, with 400 micrograms being the safe upper limit, you only need a few Brazil nuts to get more than enough! Keep this in mind because too much selenium can cause death from low blood pressure and heart failure, but this would be caused by taking more than a gram of this nutrient. For this reason, supplementation is often unnecessary because you can generally get enough selenium from your diet.

Zinc

The final trace mineral on our journey is zinc, another element that is critical to the development of the brain in children. In adults, zinc strengthens the membranes of neurons by helping convert essential fatty acids into the form that they take in the membranes. Additionally, it supports antioxidants, and it helps our brains form new neural pathways, which is essential to learning.

Zinc is concentrated in the hippocampus of the brain, where the majority of learning and memory is initiated. It helps in the creation of the neurotransmitters serotonin and melatonin, which are essential to mood regulation and sleep. Finally, it is also necessary to help rid the brain of excess lead, which is very damaging to the function of neurons.

Low levels of zinc might cause damage to brain cells, as well as depression, mood instability, and hyperactivity. Zinc deficiency has also been shown to have a relationship with psychiatric disorders like schizophrenia and severe anxiety.

Conversely, too much zinc in certain parts of the brain has been linked to Alzheimer's disease. This link may not be a result of dietary zinc, however, as zinc can sometimes be redistributed in the brain when it is injured. That said, for the most part, it would be extremely difficult to get too much zinc from the diet.

Animal sources of zinc include shellfish, meat, eggs, and dairy products. You can also find sources of zinc in pecans, Brazil nuts, peanuts, peas, rye, oats, almonds, ginger root, pumpkin seeds, sunflower seeds, and legumes such as lentils.

This is the end of our tour of essential minerals for brain function. By now, your brain is likely spinning from the alphabet soup of vitamins and minerals that you have learned about in the last two chapters. However, it does not need to be confusing. You may have noticed that certain foods were mentioned as sources of many different neuroprotective vitamins and minerals including whole grains, legumes, nuts, green leafy vegetables, pumpkin seeds, meat, fish, dairy products, and eggs. So, instead of letting yourself get overwhelmed by all of the different nutrients your brain needs, focus on the foods that have as many of these nutrients as possible. Your brain (and your budget) will thank you!

Next, we'll discuss the role that whole grains and other complex carbohydrates play in protecting your brain.

10

WHOLE GRAINS AND COMPLEX CARBS

RECENTLY, PEOPLE HAVE VIEWED CARBOHYDRATES AS BEING THE "BAD guys" when it comes to the overall health of our diets. From the prevalence of low-carbohydrate diets to the recent witch hunt against gluten, a protein commonly found in wheat, it seems that the general population has gotten the idea that carbohydrates are bad for our health.

However, the value of all carbohydrates should not be overlooked, especially when it comes to brain health. Although we should certainly be cautious of some carbohydrates, there are certain other carbs that are essential to protecting our cognitive functions. To be specific, beneficial carbohydrates come in the form of whole grains and complex carbohydrates.

Glucose and Brain Function

You may recall, from Chapter 7, that the brain is incapable of breaking down fat for energy. Although the rest of the body may use fat for energy, all fat in the brain is used for maintaining its structure. You may also recall that our brains use approximately 20 percent of our caloric intake. So, where is all of that energy coming from, if not from fat? The answer is glucose. Glucose is the go-to source of energy for the body's cells; however, since the brain cannot break down fat, it ends up using a disproportionate amount of our overall sugar intake. Of all the sugar that our bodies use for energy, approximately half of this energy goes to feeding the hungry brain.

Although the brain is capable of using other sources of energy in cases of extreme energy deprivation, glucose remains its primary and most effective source of energy. If you have ever followed a diet that emphasizes extreme restriction of sugar, you may have noticed that your thinking seemed slow, that you became irritable, and that you might have even suffered from short-term memory loss. All of these negative effects of sugar restriction are because the brain craves glucose for peak performance.

Glycemic Index (GI)

The key to providing your brain with enough glucose to function while still eating a nutritious diet is to find this sugar in healthy sources. Your best bet is to be conscious of the *glycemic index* of the carbohydrates you consume. Glycemic index, or GI, is a measurement that tells you how quickly your foods will be broken down into glucose, thereby affecting your levels of blood sugar. High GI-number foods are digested quickly, which can lead to quick blood sugar spikes followed by periods of low blood sugar. Conversely, foods that have a low GI number are digested more slowly which can lead to a steadier source of fuel for the brain and a reduction in harmful sugar spikes and crashes. We'll discuss the detrimental effects of high blood sugar later on, in Chapter 13.

Whole Grains

When it comes to grains, low GI numbers can be found in complex carbohydrates, which take longer to break down due to the presence of fiber. Fiber ultimately slows the digestion of food, leading to a more gradual release of energy in the form of glucose. High fiber grains are whole grain sources, such as whole wheat berries, quinoa, barley, rye, whole oats, millet, rice (especially brown rice), sorghum, and buckwheat; each of these grains can be prepared by cooking and eating as a side dish or as a base to any main dish. If you remember from Chapter 6, both quinoa and buckwheat provide a complete protein source, and others can be served with a legume such as black beans, lentils, or peas, to provide a dish with all 9 essential amino acids.

You can also find bread and cereal products made with 100 percent whole grains, whether they are made from whole wheat or any other grains mentioned in this section. Flour made from these whole grains is also available for your baking needs, and these serve as more nutritious (lower GI, higher fiber) alternatives to refined white flour. You may recall from the previous two chapters that whole grains are mentioned as rich sources of many brain-essential vitamins and minerals.

Fruits and Vegetables

Many fruits and vegetables are also wonderful sources of healthy carbohydrates. As with grains, those that have a low to moderate GI index number have a lot of fiber in them. Fruits that fall in this range include strawberries, blueberries, nectarines, grapes, oranges, grapefruit, bananas, cherries, pears, and kiwi. Vegetables that fall into this category include sweet potatoes, carrots, broccoli, cauliflower, zucchini, tomatoes, and celery. Like the whole grains with low GI numbers, many of these fruits and vegetables have the added benefits of neuroprotective vitamins and minerals. It is no coincidence that many types of foods contain multiple nutrients that are necessary for optimal brain function and reducing your risk of dementia.

Fiber

Another technique for lowering the overall glycemic index number of your meal is to add sources of fiber to your meals. Although they do not contain much glucose, dark green leafy vegetables are a great addition to any dish or meal because they contribute fiber, thereby slowing the digestive process and reducing blood sugar spikes.

An added benefit of eating fibrous foods is that they help to fight inflammation. Within the body, fiber from foods contributes to the synthesis of fatty acid that helps reduce inflammation. Since reduced inflammation in the brain is associated with a decreased risk of developing age-related neurodegenerative diseases, fiber-rich foods certainly play many roles in regards to keeping our brains young and healthy!

Other foods that do not have much glucose but that contribute fiber to your diet are legumes like peas and beans. You probably remember other benefits of legumes that were discussed in the chapters about protein, vitamins, and minerals.

Understanding Gluten

One of the reasons that some grains have been avoided by many in recent years is the presence of the dreaded *gluten* in them. However, for most healthy people, gluten is not something that needs to be feared or avoided; it has just gotten a bad reputation due to some bad publicity. In fact, gluten is a substance that is present in many grains. On a molecular level, it is a combination of two different proteins. Each grain (like a kernel of barley or a single wheat berry) is a seed that nature made to grow into an individual new plant. Gluten is stored within the grains, along with starch, to help supply nutrients to a tiny seedling when the grains begin to grow into tiny new plants.

Gluten has gained a lot of publicity lately due to a something called *Celiac disease*. With this genetic disorder, eating gluten prompts the body's immune system to attack cells of the small intestine, prompting extremely serious issues with digestion and other organs. Besides Celiac disease, some other people suffer from sensitivity to gluten. This sensitivity is not necessarily genetic, nor does it involve an autoimmune response. Sensitivity to gluten can lead to very uncomfortable symptoms like mental confusion, exhaustion, numbness of the extremities, digestive problems, headaches, and even joint pain.

For the approximately ten percent of the population that suffer from Celiac disease or who have a gluten sensitivity, grains that contain gluten should be avoided at all costs. These grains are wheat (including various varieties of wheat, like spelt and bulgar), rye, triticale, barley, and oats. However, these people can still enjoy grains like millet, sorghum, corn, rice, quinoa, and buckwheat.

For the rest of the population who do not suffer any ill effects from consuming gluten-containing products, all whole grains are up for grabs. The brain-healthy diets outlined in Chapter 3 include plentiful whole grains because of the myriad benefits to the brain and cardiovascular system. Of course, it is still important to balance these carbohydrates with healthy protein, fruits, vegetables, and (mostly good) fats.

This is the end of the major categories of foods that benefit the brain. However, there are still a few other foods that are worth mentioning. You may be surprised by a couple of them, because you may have never imagined that they could be good for you!

11

TASTY LITTLE EXTRAS

BESIDES THE HEALTHY FOODS THAT YOU HAVE ALREADY LEARNED about, there are a few other categories that you should know about. These "bonus foods" can add a little fun and extra flavor to your diet, while still being extremely important for protecting your brain.

Eggs

We have already discussed eggs a few times in this guide because they are great sources of protein and provide lots of brain-healthy vitamins and minerals. However, they are worth mentioning one more time because of one very important component: *choline.* Choline is an essential nutrient to the brain because it is needed to make acetylcholine, one of the important neurotransmitters used for communication between neurons.

Choline is not only found in eggs, but eggs are one of the richest sources of this nutrient. The recommended daily allowance of choline is 550 mg per day for men and 425 mg per day for women. For example, one egg yolk contains a whopping 115 mg of choline. So, while it's not the best idea to eat 4 or 5 eggs every day, eating them once or twice a week can help contribute to your healthy choline intake. Other foods that contain choline include dairy sources, beef liver, and cruciferous vegetables like broccoli and cauliflower. As always, you should talk to a doctor before considering taking a choline supplement.

Caffeine

According to various studies, when consumed in moderate amounts, coffee and tea can boost your short-term and possibly your long-term memory abilities. Particularly when consumed directly after learning new information, drinking one or two cups of coffee helps you to retain that new information. But, what about any long-term benefits of caffeine?

Well, some studies have shown that consuming coffee is linked to a significantly reduced risk of developing Alzheimer's disease. However, researchers still need to determine whether this association is just coincidental or if caffeine does actually have neuroprotective qualities. For example, there is evidence that caffeine has anti-inflammatory properties, and, as you have learned, reducing inflammation is one of the keys to avoiding Alzheimer's. There is still no definite answer, but for now, it seems that you can continue to sip on a daily cup or two of coffee.

However, be sure not to overdo it on the caffeine as another lifestyle factor that contributes to good brain health is consistently getting enough sleep. Too much caffeine late in the day is disruptive to your sleep cycle and can eventually lead to an increased rate of brain cell damage.

Dark Chocolate

Chocolate lovers can breathe easy knowing that their favorite treat is allowed to remain in their diet in small quantities. For example, raw cocoa contains powerful antioxidants called flavanols that are important to the brain. Specifically, these antioxidants can help to increase blood flow toward the brain, which leads to better memory and improves other mental skills. Additionally, studies have concluded that eating a small amount of dark chocolate every day can help prevent neurodegenerative diseases.

Don't race out and buy pounds of your favorite candy bars, though. This is because dark chocolate, specifically, has more benefits than milk chocolate, which has less cocoa and more sugar. Therefore, the fewer sugary additives (like nougat or caramel), the better, though it's all right to enjoy dark chocolate that has a few nuts in it because these are healthy for your brain as well. Just a little dark chocolate is plenty for enjoying health benefits without consuming too many unnecessary calories.

Red Wine

You probably noticed that all of the diets outlined in Chapter 3 specifically mentioned a daily glass of red wine as an acceptable beverage. The reason for including this in heart-and-brain-healthy diets is that it has a high concentration of the antioxidant resveratrol. Research has shown that this antioxidant can help to repair the blood-brain barrier and reduce inflammation in the brain, thus helping to prevent dementia and other neurodegenerative conditions.

Benefits from red wine are derived when it is consumed in low to moderate amounts, and health experts recommend no more than one or two small glasses daily. Ultimately, however, if you do not drink, there is no need to start as resveratrol is also present in red grapes, peanuts, pistachios, blueberries, and cranberries.

Berries

Besides the resveratrol mentioned above, very high concentrations of other antioxidants can be found in berries like blueberries, strawberries, raspberries, and blackberries. The antioxidant levels in these tiny but powerful fruits are so high that they have been shown to help improve the quality of communication between neurons in the brain. They may also help to prevent inflammation that can lead to neurodegeneration.

Other fruits with high levels of antioxidants are those with dark skins like plums, blackberries, and cherries.

Herbs and Spices

In terms of flavorful additions to your diet, several herbs and spices have been associated with better brain health and possible decreased risks of Alzheimer's disease:

- *Sage* – may improve memory abilities
- *Turmeric* – may have anti-inflammatory properties and may help to prevent the buildup of brain plaques associated with Alzheimer's
- *Gingko Biloba* – may help to improve cognitive abilities and slow the progression of dementia
- *Ashwagandha* – may inhibit the formation of Alzheimer's plaques and act as an antioxidant
- *Ginseng* – has anti-inflammatory chemicals and may reduce levels of beta-amyloid in the brain (precursor to plaques)
- *Gotu kola* – may have antioxidant properties; often taken to decrease "brain fog"
- *Lemon balm* – improves cognition and may help to decrease insomnia and anxiety
- *Rosemary* – may improve memory abilities
- *Cinnamon* – contains antioxidant properties
- *Curry* – may help destroy beta-amyloid plaques or slow their formation

None of the "extras" mentioned in this chapter are harmful to your health unless you overindulge in any of them! So, enjoy experimenting with flavors and sweet treats that may benefit your brain.

In the next part, you'll learn about foods that you should avoid or only enjoy in limited quantities due to their potentially negative effects on your brain.

PART III

ENEMIES OF THE BRAIN

12

TRANS AND SATURATED FATS

As much as I hate to be a downer, we must discuss certain foods that can be harmful to your brain. After all, you wouldn't want to undo all the good you have done for your brain by eating unhealthy foods, would you?

The first unfortunate subject on our plate is certain fats, some of which you should eat in small quantities, and others of which you should avoid altogether.

Saturated Fats

We discussed different types of fats in Chapter 7 but only looked in-depth at the "good" fats which are mono-and-polyunsaturated fatty acids. Now, we will look at the so-called "bad" fats. *Saturated fats*, as you may recall, are long chains of carbon atoms with no double bonds. Because these fats have no double bonds, every possible place in the chain is "saturated" with hydrogen atoms. This saturation makes these fats more stable than unsaturated fats, so they tend to be in solid form at room temperature, though they do melt at high temperatures.

Sources of saturated fats include red meat like pork, beef, and lamb. Other sources include poultry (skin on) and animal products like dairy, lard, butter, cream, and full or reduced-fat milk, cheese, and yogurt; coconut oil and palm oil also have saturated fat.

Saturated fats are a necessary part of your diet in low to moderate quantities for a few different reasons. For one, they contribute to the structure of your brain, so they are especially important for still-developing babies and children. It also plays important roles in the immune system, the storage of energy, and liver health. Additionally, including a small amount of saturated fat in one meal per day is very satisfying and can even help to keep you from overeating. Saturated fat also helps maintain healthy cholesterol levels in your blood. Regarding brain health, coconut oil, in particular, has been shown to help heal neurons.

However, you can get too much of a good thing. Studies have shown that eating too much saturated fat is linked to excessive cholesterol which contributes to the danger of heart disease and vascular damage to the brain, including stroke. Research that focuses on cognitive decline has also linked the consumption of saturated fats to an increased risk of impaired memory and dementia.

You should try to get no more than 5 to 6 percent of your diet from saturated fat. So, if you eat 2,000 calories per day, that would be about 120 calories or 13 grams of saturated fat which is equivalent to about two tablespoons of butter.

If you evaluate your diet and find that you are consuming too many sources of saturated fat, consider making substitutions. For example, instead of red meat, eat fish or skinless poultry, or try your hand at some vegetarian sources of protein once a week or more (see Chapter 6 for ideas). Additionally, instead of using a lot of butter for cooking and flavoring, substitute it with cold-pressed extra virgin olive oil and seek out nonfat or low-fat versions of your favorite dairy products.

Trans Fats

In an ideal world, an ominous musical tone should sound every time we see or hear the phrase, "trans fats", to warn you of impending doom - that's how bad they are for you.

In Chapter 7, you learned that trans fats are (usually) artificially produced to extend a product's shelf life. Trans fats are made by transforming generally healthy liquid fats into solids by adding extra hydrogen atoms. In other words, unsaturated fats become artificially saturated or hydrogenated through chemical processes. In the end, these chains of fatty acids stack tightly together, and it is very difficult for your body to break them down.

In contrast to saturated fats which do have benefits in small quantities, trans fats do not carry any benefits and are best avoided altogether. In the brain, these harmful fats can increase inflammation and reduce the amount of healthy Omega-3s that are produced. Trans fats have also been shown to impair memory abilities and decrease emotional stability. Modern research continues to find more and more evidence that suggests trans fat may play a role in the development of age-related cognitive decline, including Alzheimer's disease.

Trans fats can sometimes be tricky to avoid as they are found in many processed foods such as delicious, commercially baked goods. Sneaky sources of trans fat can also include salad dressings, snack foods, and fast foods. Plus, even if you look at the nutrition facts, you may be missing hidden trans fats. This is because if there is less than 0.5 g of trans fat in a serving size, manufacturers are allowed to list the trans fat content as "0", and since we rarely only eat *one* serving of anything, we could be eating up to a gram or two of this harmful fat without even knowing it! It's best to read ingredients and steer clear of hydrogenated or partially hydrogenated oils! If your brain could talk, it would thank you for doing so.

13
_____

SIMPLE CARBOHYDRATES

In Chapter 10, you learned about carbohydrates as a source of glucose, which is your brain's main source of energy. You also learned that you could get the most benefit from glucose by choosing foods that have a low Glycemic Index (GI) number, meaning that these foods are digested slowly and provide steady sources of energy. Here, we'll look at foods on the other end of the GI spectrum.

High GI Foods

The opposite of complex carbohydrates with low GI numbers is simple carbohydrates, including refined sugar. Simple carbohydrates break down into glucose quickly, leading to rapid rises and subsequent drops in your blood sugar levels.

Sudden blood sugar spikes are harmful to your body in many ways. If you eat a lot of high GI index foods on a regular basis throughout many years, you can potentially develop type 2 diabetes where your body will not be able to use insulin to get blood sugar into your cells for energy. Additionally, glucose then builds up in your blood. High levels of blood sugar damage the body in many ways, leading to symptoms like extreme thirst, excessive urination, and fatigue. More serious complications of consistently high blood sugar are poor circulation, extreme nerve damage and infections, blurry vision, digestive problems, kidney failure, heart attack, and stroke.

Because high blood sugar affects circulation, it directly affects the amount of oxygen and other nutrients that reach the brain. Poor circulation to the brain can cause problems with memory and other cognitive functions and increase the risk of Alzheimer's disease or other forms of dementia. Scientific research has shown that poor memory and risks of dementia are associated with high blood sugar even in people that don't have diabetes.

Foods that are natural but have higher GI numbers include white rice and white potatoes. These are broken down quickly by your body and can lead to rapid spikes and drops in blood sugar levels. Additionally, fruit juices and honey have moderate GI numbers and should be consumed in moderation. Besides natural foods, many processed foods are high on the GI and include processed cereals and bread that are produced from refined flour, as well as cookies, donuts, pasta, and crackers (that are not made with whole grains). Beverages like sweet tea or sugary sodas are also loaded with simple sugars such as high-fructose corn syrup and thus rank high on the GI scale.

Risks of Too Much Sugar in the Diet

Beyond choosing foods with low GI, we should also be wary of simply consuming too much sugar in our diets. Even if we can (generally) maintain healthy blood sugar levels and never develop diabetes, excessive consumption of sugar is still damaging to the brain. Unfortunately, eating too much sugar is a common issue, especially in Western and American diet. Experts recommend consuming no more than 25 grams of added sugar per day for women and 37.5 grams for men every day, yet most Americans consume more than 2 to 3 times that amount!

Consuming too much sugar over a short period of time can cause depression and anxiety due to variations in blood sugar levels and the effect that these fluctuations have on hormones and neurotransmitters. Additionally, excessive sugar in the diet has been linked to the rapid aging of cells throughout the body, including the brain. A reduction of cognitive functions can occur as the body is less able to use insulin efficiently as a result of eating too much sugar.

The reason behind these negative impacts of sugar on the brain may have to do with a chemical called *Brain-Derived Neurotrophic Factor (BDNF)*. BDNF is produced in the brain, but scientific research has shown that too much sugar decreases its production. Less BDNF interferes significantly with our ability to learn and remember information; low levels of this chemical have also been linked with dementia and depression.

What's the Solution?

Before you decide to switch to diet sodas that are full of artificial sweeteners, you should know that consumption of these calorie-free sweeteners has also been linked to an increased risk of dementia. So, you would be better off eliminating soda altogether and reaching for unsweetened iced tea or water, which can be flavored with numerous fruits as described in Chapter 5.

Instead of sugary junk food and baked goods, try filling up on wholesome, satisfying foods instead. Getting the right amounts of healthy fats, protein, and carbohydrates in your diet is generally very satisfying and unlikely to leave you craving candy bars and cookies. Of course, it is fine to enjoy the occasional treat, but try to limit these for your best chance of keeping your brain sharp for decades to come.

14

ALCOHOL

Even though you have learned of the benefits of the occasional (or even daily) glass of red wine, a word of caution is necessary when it comes to alcohol. Although it may be tempting to reach for a second or third glass of wine, research shows that long-term, excessive alcohol consumption can be just as damaging to your brain as too much sugar or trans fats, if not more so.

The Long-Term Negative Effects of Alcohol

You may have heard of people experiencing blackouts from drinking too much alcohol, or you may have even experienced one or two of these yourself. Blackouts are periods of time in which a person cannot remember certain details (or anything at all) from a certain period of time. Blackouts tend to happen after a person has consumed enough alcohol in a short period to increase their blood alcohol level rapidly. Ultimately, blackouts are indicators of the effects of excessive alcohol consumption on the brain.

The brains of alcoholic men and women who drank heavily for many years have been studied via computer imaging and brain scans. Indications of brain damage, such as shrinkage in the overall size of the brain, were common in these subjects, particularly among women. Additional symptoms of prolonged heavy drinking can be poor memory, a reduction of other cognitive functions, and reduced blood flow to the brain, eventually leading to vascular dementia or stroke.

Besides directly damaging the brain, prolonged heavy alcohol consumption can lead to a deficiency in thiamin or B1 due to the inability of an alcoholic's body to absorb this vitamin. As you learned in Chapter 8, thiamin is essential to brain function, and deficiencies in this nutrient can cause poor memory, confusion, and even permanent brain damage.

Some of the damage done by alcoholism to the brain has been shown to be reversible, but complete cognitive recovery may not be possible. Still, many recovering alcoholics have enjoyed improved memory abilities and an overall clearing of "brain fog."

Finally, if you have found that you are unable to stop drinking on your own, or if you cannot stop drinking any time you start, you may have a problem. If that is the case, it is vital to the future function of your brain, and to your life that you seek help from a qualified specialist.

CONCLUSION

Thanks for making it through to the end of *Brain Food Diet: Cognitive Decline and Alzheimer's Disease Reversed with Anti-aging Longevity Diet.* We hope that it was informative and able to provide you with the tools you need to achieve your goals of sustaining the health of your brain for a lifetime.

The next step is to go shopping for the foods in this book! Now is the time to start preventing dementia and reversing the signs of age-related cognitive decline. Write down a shopping list that includes wild-caught salmon, extra virgin olive oil (cold-pressed, of course), nuts, beans, whole grains, and plenty of different fruits and vegetables. Don't forget some red wine and dark chocolate too! While you're at it, bring a water bottle and always remember to hydrate, hydrate, hydrate.

If you follow the nutritional guidelines outlined in this book, you, your friends, and your family members may be surprised at how sharp your memory remains for the rest of your life, even into your 80s and beyond. The people in Okinawa, Loma Linda, Bulgaria, and Sardinia have discovered the secret to aging gracefully, and now that secret is in your hands as well. So, what are you waiting for? It's time to act and start eating your way to better brain health.

Finally, if you found this book useful in any way, a review on Amazon is always appreciated!

Made in the USA
Lexington, KY
12 July 2019